Plant Pathology
Fundamentals and Applications

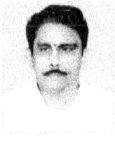

Prof. Dr. B. Srinivasulu obtained his M.Sc. (Ag.) Plant Pathology and Ph.D (Plant Pathology) from Tamil Nadu Agricultural University, Coimbatore. Recipient of IDRC, Canada fellowship for the Doctoral programme. He has been actively associated in research and development of Plant Pathology since 31 years in his capacity as Research Associate at ICRISAT, as Scientist, Senior Scientist and Principal Scientist at ANGRAU and as Principal Scientist at Dr.YSRHU.

Dr. B.Srinivasulu is a recipient of Gold Medal (1999) and prestigious awards – Dr.D.Bap Reddy Memorial award (2004), PLACROSYM – XVI award (2004), AAU Best Research award (2004), NRCOP Best Research award (2005), Dr.C.S.Venkataram Memorial award (2006), Biotechnology and Pharmacy award (2007), Uddaraju Ananda Raju Foundation Award – 2012, 'State Best Officer' Ugadi Puraskaram from Govt. of Andhra Pradesh – 2012, International prestigious Sardar Patel Award – 2013.

He has written 6 books, chapters in 6 books, 30 bulletins and published 123 research and 105 popular articles.

Dr.B.Srinivasulu is currently Registrar, Dr.Y.S.R. Horticultural University, Venkataramannagudem, Andhra Pradesh.

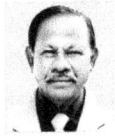

Prof. M. Rajamannar obtained his M.Sc. (Ag.) from GBPUAT, Pantnagar and Ph.D. from IARI. He was awarded Gold Medal for Ph. D. Programme at IARI, New Delhi. He joined APAU (presently ANGRAU) in 1976 as Research Assistant and Retired as Principal Scientist (Plant Pathology) at A. P. Rice Research Institute, Maruteru in 2007. Greater part of his research career was spent on Tatipaka and Ganoderma basal stem rot of coconut. He was associated with the work related to the phytoplasmal etiology of Tatipaka disease and integrated management of both the diseases. He has published 35 research articles in national and international journals and chapters in books and jointly authored technical bulletins published by CPCRI, AICRP on Palms and ANGRAU. He also served as Professor at Agricultural College, Naira and taught Plant Pathology. He attended more than 30 National and International seminars, symposia, workshops etc. and presented papers. He served as selection committee member and external examiner for several institutions. He was a member of several committees on coconut and oil palm and disaster management teams of CPCRI and ANGRAU. His expertise extends over diagnosis of field problems to modern techniques like light and fluorescent microscopy, electron microscopy, ELISA, immunoblotting, ultracentrifugation, electrophoresis etc. in the laboratory. He has vast experience over diseases of rice, coconut, oil palm, banana, cocoa, pepper, papaya and several other crops and their integrated management.

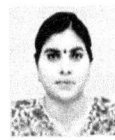

Mrs. T. Nagalakshmi obtained her M.Sc. (Ag.) in Plant Pathology from Agricultural College, Andhra Pradesh Agricultural University, Bapatla. She worked as Scientist (Plant Pathology) at ICRISAT from 2005 to 2008. Attended CMMYT International Workshop at Nairobi, Kenya. She has written 10 bulletins and published 15 articles. She is currently working as Scientist (Plant Pathology), Horticultural Research Station, Dr. Y.S.R. Horticultural University at Anantharajupeta, Andhra Pradesh.

Plant Pathology
Fundamentals and Applications

— With Classical Examples of Horticultural Crops —

Prof. Dr. B. Srinivasulu

Prof. M. Rajamannar

Mrs. T. Nagalakshmi

2017

Daya Publishing House®

A Division of

Astral International Pvt. Ltd.

New Delhi – 110 002

Cataloging in Publication Data--DK
  Courtesy: D.K. Agencies (P) Ltd. <docinfo@dkagencies.com>

  Srinivasulu, B., author.
  Plant pathology : fundamentals and applications : with classical examples of horticultural crops / authors, Prof. Dr. B. Srinivasulu, Prof. M. Rajamannar, Mrs. T. Nagalakshmi.
        pages cm
        Includes bibliographical references and index.
        ISBN 978-93-86071-76-7 (International Edition)

        1. Horticultural crops--Diseases and pests.   I. Rajamannar, M., author. II. Nagalakshmi, T., author. III. Title.
  SB608.H83S65 2017   DDC 635.92   23

Published by   : **Daya Publishing House®**
                                A Division of
                                Astral International Pvt. Ltd.
                                – ISO 9001:2015 Certified Company –
                                4736/23, Ansari Road, Darya Ganj
                                New Delhi-110 002
                                Ph. 011-43549197, 23278134
                                E-mail: info@astralint.com
                                Website: www.astralint.com

Preface

This textbook "Plant Pathology: Fundamentals and Applications" is being brought out to fulfill the need for a comprehensive source of information on Plant Pathology to undergraduate students of Agriculture. Though several textbooks are available, many are either exhaustive, or deal with a particular aspect of the subject or costly. An undergraduate student requires to grab information from different sources within a limited time for his preparation to the subject. This causes lot of pressure on the performance of the student.

The main objective of bringing out this book to provide all main ingredients of Plant Pathology briefly at one place. As such, the book has been conveniently into 17 units. Each chapter included needed illustrations, examples with photographs for better understanding. Keeping the difficulties of the students in mind, we have made all effort to furnish not only a simple, authentic, classical account but also recent advance s in understanding the subject and its implications on present day Agriculture. Despite all the efforts we made, there might be some shortcomings of different opacities in the book. We regret for all such shortcomings, in advance. We whole heartedly welcome all constructive suggestions from the readers to improve upon in further editions.

While preparing the manuscripts, we used information from different sources including internet, which have been included in the references. We thank to all those who permitted to use the information including the photographs. We wish to state that all the information used in this book is meant for educating the students.

B. Srinivasulu
M. Rajamannar
T. Nagalakshmi

Contents

1
Introduction

Phytopathology (*phyton* = plant; *pathos* = suffering; *logos* = knowledge), in other words, Plant Pathology is a branch of agricultural, botanical or biological science which deals with the etiology, symptoms/damage, resulting losses and control of plant diseases.

What is a Disease?

☆ Disease can be defined as a physiological disorder or structural abnormality that is deleterious to the plant or to any of its parts or products that reduces their economic values. (Stakman and Harrar, 1957); or

☆ Any disturbance brought about by a living entity or non-living agents or environmental factors which interfere with manufacture, translocation or utilization of food, minerals and water in such a way that the affected plant changes in appearance with or without much loss in yield that of a normal healthy plant of the same variety. (Agrios G.N. 1978); or

☆ In short, it is anything that affects the health of the plants hindering their normal growth and yield.

Objectives of Plant Pathology

The science of *Phytopathology* has four major objectives:

1. To study the living, non-living, and environmental causes of plant diseases;

2. To study the mechanisms of disease development;

3. To study the interaction between the plant and pathogen; and

4. To develop methods for controlling/managing diseases and reducing the losses caused by them.

Groups of Plant Pathogens

Common biotic causes of diseases in plants belong to Fungi, Bacteria, Viruses, Viroids, Algae, Fastidious vascular bacteria (RLO's), Phytoplasmas (MLO's), Spiroplasmas, Protozoa, Nematodes and Phanerogamic parasites.

The biotic agents are categorized into prokaryotes and eukaryotes based on the nuclear organization and other physiological processes involved in their growth and development. While bacteria, phytoplasmas, protozoa, etc., belong to prokaryota; fungi, nematodes, algae and phanerogamic parasites come under eukaryota. The main differences between these two groups have been tabulated here.

		Prokaryotes	Eukaryotes
a)	Size	1-10 microns	10-100 microns
b)	Complexity	Unicellular, rarely small clusters or filaments	Sometimes unicellular; more often multicellular
c)	Membrane bound organelles	None (mesosome is in folding of cytoplasmic membrane)	Nuclei, mitochondria, chloroplasts, lysosomes, endoplasmic reticulum, golgi and vacuoles
d)	Nucleus	No	Yes
e)	Chromosomes	Single and circular	Usually several and linear
f)	Introns and Exons	Occasionally	Frequent
g)	Histones	No	Yes
h)	Ploidy	Haploid	Diploid
i)	Mitosis and Meiosis	Absent	Present
j)	Sexual reproduction	None, or unidirectional from donor to recipient	Usually, involves fusion of haploid gametes
k)	Ribosomes	70s (50s + 30s sub-units)	80s (60s + 40s) in cytoplasm; (mitochondria and chloroplasts have prokaryotic ribosomes)
l)	Cytoskeleton	Absent	Microtubules and microfilaments
m)	Cell wall	Usually present, contains peptidoglycan	Absent in animals; present in fungi (chitin) and plants (cellulose)
n)	Motility	Simple, prokaryotic, flagella, gliding motion	Complex "9+2" flagella or cilia with centrioles
o)	Endocytosis and cytoplasmic streaming	Absent	Present
p)	Differentiation	Usually absent	Cells differentiate to form tissues and organs
q)	Energy metabolism	Many diverse pathways in various bacteria	Glycolysis in cytoplasm, Krebs Cycle and ETC in mitochondria
r)	Oxygen	Aerobic and/or anaerobic	Usually aerobic
s)	Sterols	Usually absent	Used as hormones and in plasma membrane

1. Fungi

Eukaryotic, spore-bearing, achlorophyllous, generally reproduce sexually and asexually, filamentous branched somatic structures, typically surrounded by cell walls containing chitin or cellulose or both, saprophytic, pathogenic or symbionts absorptive nutrition.

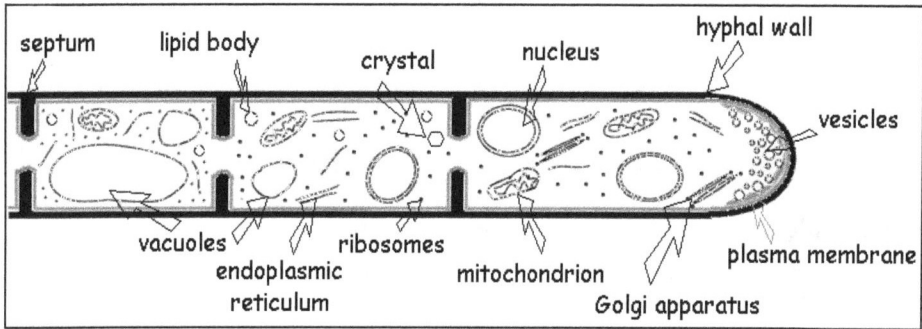

Figure 1: Structure of a Typical Fungal Tip.

2. Bacteria

Prokaryotic, rigid, unicellular, free of true chlorophyll, generally devoid of any photosynthetic pigment, most commonly multiplying asexually by simple transverse fission.

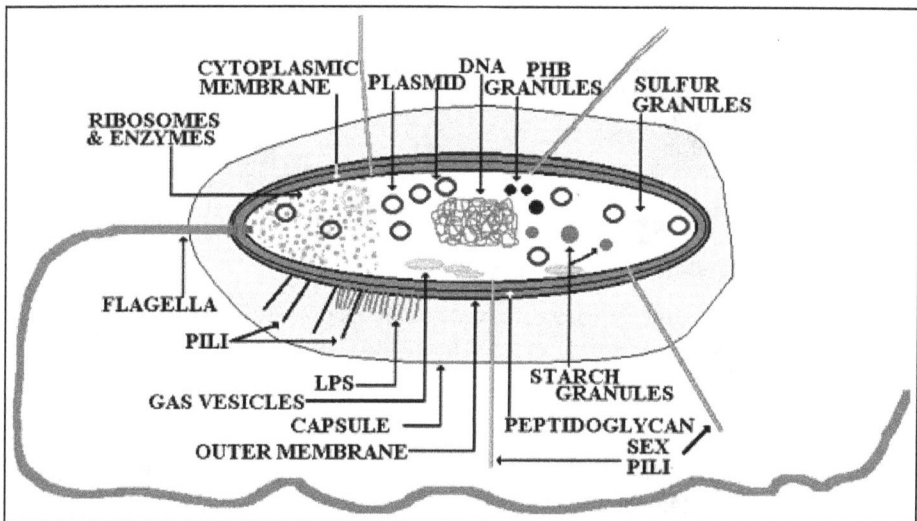

Figure 2: A Typical Bacterial Cell.

3. Fastidious Vascular Bacteria (Rickettssia like organisms, RLOs)

Similar to bacteria in most respects but cannot be grown on routine bacteriological media and needs complex medium for its growth.

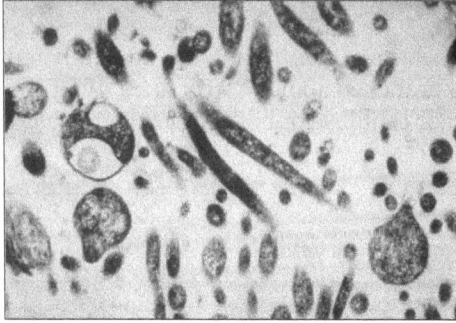

Figure 3: Typical RLOs in Host Cells.

4. Phytoplasma (MLO's) (Non-helical mollicutes)

Prokaryotic, pleomorphic, wall-less prokaryotic micro-organisms, infect plants and cannot yet to be grown in culture.

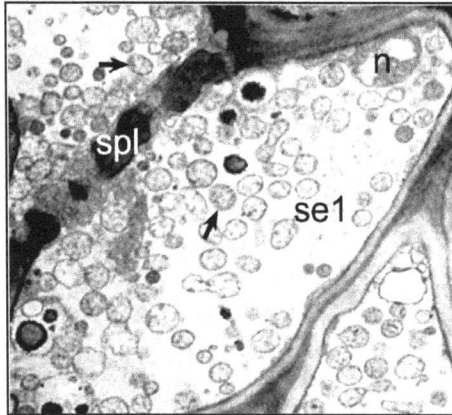

Figure 4: Phytoplasmas in Phloem Sieve Tubes of Host Plants.

5. Spiroplasma (Helical mollicutes)

Prokaryotic, helical, wall-less micro-organisms, present in phloem of diseased plants, often helical in culture, thought to be a kind of mycoplasma, can be cultured on artificial medium.

6. Virus/Virion

Sub-microscopic, potentially pathogenic obligate parasites, consisting of mainly nucleic acid and protein, multiplies only intra-cellularly.

7. Viroid (Naked nucleic acid or virus without protein coat)

Smallest known plant pathogens with low molecular weight ribonucleic acid (ssRNA), without protein coat, replicate themselves, cause disease only in plants.

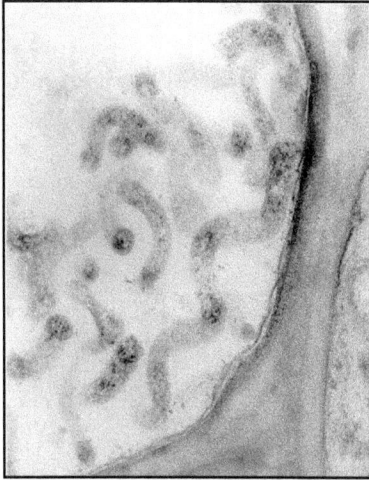

Figure 5: Corn Stunt Spiroplasma in Host Cell.

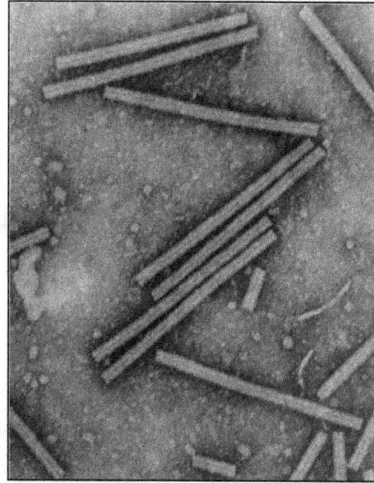

Figure 6: Rod-shaped Virus Particles of Tobacco Misaic *tobamovirus*.

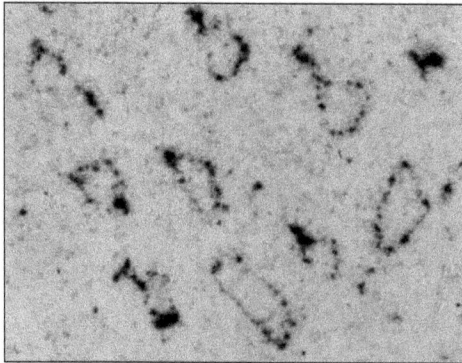

Figure 7: Potato Spindle Tuber Viroid seen in Electron Microscope (EM).

8. Protozoa

Microscopic, non-photosynthetic, eukaryotic, flagellate, motile, single-celled animals.

9. Algae (Few algae mainly green algae)

Eukaryotic, photosynthetic, uni-, or multi-cellular organisms, containing chlorophyll, causing plant diseases.

10. Phanerogamic Parasites

These flowering parasitic plants damage the host plants through exhaustion of nutrients and sometimes through restriction in growth of the plant. Few of them produce toxins.

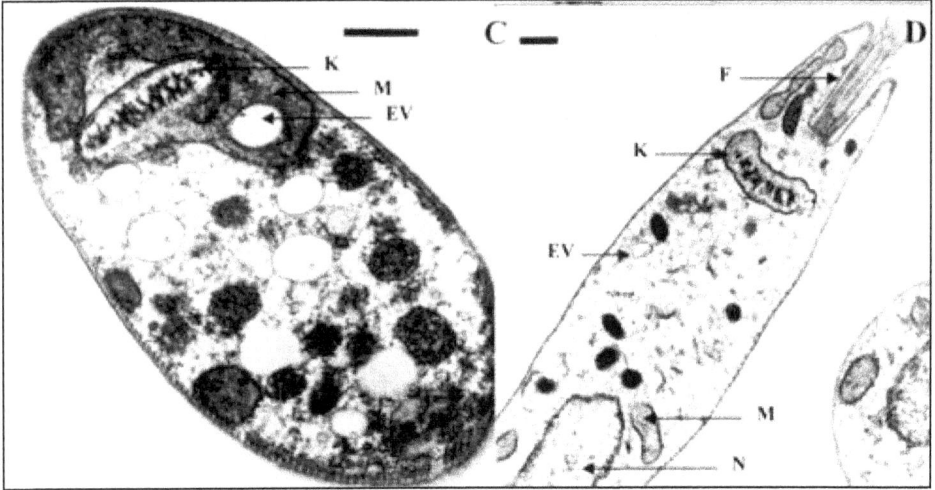

Figure 8: Structure of Plant Parasitic Protozoa.

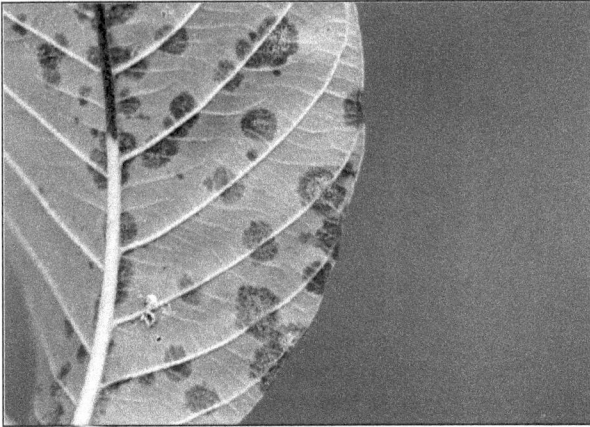

Figure 9: Algal Parasite Infection on Guava Leaf Causing Red Rust.

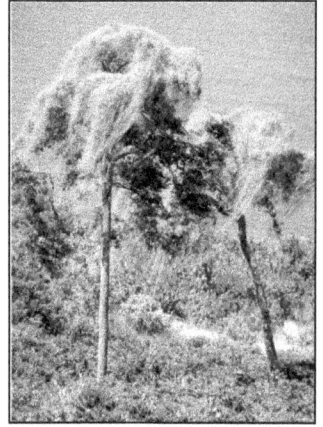

Figure 10: *Cassytha filiformis* on Trees.

Economic Importance of Plant Diseases

Plant diseases are important because of the losses or sufferings they cause. The loss can occur in the field or in the store and at anytime between sowing and consumption of the produce. In the history of mankind plant diseases have been connected with a number of important events that caused great sufferings and also changed the life style of people of a community or even a country.

1. Late blight of potato, caused by *Phytophthora infestans*, is a famous example of what a plant disease can do to change the course of history. In 1845, this disease destroyed the potato crop of Ireland which was the staple food of the population. In Ireland alone the populations of 8 million was

reduced to 6 million. There was migration of large population to other lands including the North American continent. This single disease forced man to realise the importance of plant diseases.

2. In 1878-1882, the wine industry in France was threatened due to epiphytotic destruction of Grapes by the downy mildew fungus, *Plasmopara viticola*.

3. In 1867, *Hemileia vastatrix* (the coffee rust pathogen) attacked coffee plantations in Sri Lanka (fka Ceylon) and the export of coffee was reduced by 93 per cent and the area under coffee has been replaced with tea plantations.

4. In 1910, "Panama Wilt" of Banana occurred on a large scale in Panama and Surinam. Banana cultivation was abandoned in several parts of Australia also, because of the severity of panama wilt disease.

5. In 1930, the entire banana industry in central and south America was threatened with extinction due to 'Sigatoka leaf spot' caused by *Mycosphaerella musicola*.

6. In Argentina and Brazil, large scale occurrence of 'Tristeza' disease ruined the citrus industry.

7. Nematode: According to Seinhorst (1965) – Damage caused by nematodes is very significant. They slowly declined the orchard trees like Apple, citrus, walnut, cherry and prune in many countries due to Ecto-and endoparasitic nematodes.

2
History of Plant Pathology

The earliest record on the occurrence of plant diseases can be traced back to about 1500 B.C. in Vedas mentioning plant diseases and their control. Surapal, an ancient Indian Scholar, wrote first book 'Vrikshayurvada' in Sanskrit on plant life that included plant diseases and plant protection from internal and external diseases. There are also references on blast diseases, mildews in the Old Testament (The Bible). An annual festival, 'Robigalia', used to be celebrated in Rome to ward of the crops from rust disease. Theophrastus (370-276 B.C.) studied and wrote about the diseases of trees, cereals and legumes based on his observations. In 857 A.D., the first serious outbreak of ergotism was recorded in the Rhine Valley. It struck the peasants and killed thousands of people.

In 1675 the Dutch worker, Leeuwenhoek, developed the first microscope and in 1683 he described bacteria seen with his microscope. When these micro-organisms were seen associated with diseased plants it was suggested that the disease, however, was not due to these organisms but was of spontaneous origin.

Pier (Pietro) Antonio Micheli (1679-1737)

In 1729, the Italian botanist Pier Antonio Micheli described many new genera of fungi and illustrated their reproductive structures. He also noted that when placed on freshly cut slices of melon, these structures grew and produced the same kind of fungus that had produced them. He proposed, therefore, that fungi arise from their own spores rather than spontaneously, but because the "spontaneous generation" theory was so imbedded in people's minds, nobody believed Micheli's evidence. He published a book called *"Nova Plantorum Genera"*.

Needham

In 1743, this English scientist observed nematodes inside small, abnormally rounded wheat kernels (ear cockle of wheat), but he too failed to show or suggest that they were the cause of the problem.

Mathieu Tillet (1714-1791)

The Frenchman Tillet, working with smutted wheat, showed that he could increase the number of wheat plants developing covered smut by dusting wheat kernels before planting with smut dust, *i.e.*, with a smut spores. He also noted that he could reduce the number of smutted wheat plants produced by treating the smut-treated kernels with copper sulfate. Tillet too, however, did not interpret his experiments properly and, instead of concluding that wheat smut is an infectious plant disease, he believed that it was a poisonous substance contained in the smut dust, rather than the living spores and fungus coming from them that caused the disease. In 1755, he published a paper titled Bunt or stinking smut of wheat established role of fungi in plant disease showed contagious nature of wheat bunt suggested control-seed treatment with salt and lime.

Benedict Prevost (1755-1819)

Another Frenchman repeated both the inoculation experiments and those in which the seeds were treated with copper sulfate, as done by Tillet, and he obtained the same results. In addition, Prevost observed smut spores from untreated and treated wheat seed under the microscope and noticed that those from untreated seed germinated and grew whereas those from treated seed failed to germinate. He, therefore, concluded correctly that it was the smut spores that caused the smut disease in wheat and that the reduced number of smutted wheat plants derived from copper sulfate. He was the first person to prove micro-organism as cause of plant disease and first proved *Tilletia caries* as causal organism of wheat bunt. Described germination of bunt spores, discovered life cycle of bunt fungus and also demonstrated control-seed treatment with $CuSO_4$ solution, studied fungicidal and fungistatic properties of chemicals and published classic-paper 'Memoir on immediate cause on bunt of wheat' in 1807. Prevost's conclusions were not accepted by French Academy of Sciences, which strongly supported the theory of Spontaneous Generations.

Christiaan Hendrik Persoon (1761-1836)

Native of South Africa, basically medical doctor laid foundation for mycological taxonomy. He described and named *Puccinia graminis* in 1794. He published a book '*Synopsis Methodica Fungorum*' in 1801 which was considered as one of the starting point for nomenclature of fungi. The book formed the basis for nomenclature of Uredinales, Ustilaginales, Gasteromycetes. First established a useable system for classification of fungi, developed herbarium at Lei den (The Netherlands) later taken up by the Dutch government in 1822. He published '*Mycologia Europaea*', but sold it to Dutch government because of poverty.

Elias Magnus Fries (1794-1878)

This Sweden taxonomist professor of botany at University of Sweden specialised in *Agaricus and* was regarded as '**Linnaeus of mycology**' or '**Father of systematic mycology**', through his book entitled "*Systema Mycologicum*" *in* 8 volumes written in 1821. This is considered as the starting date for nomenclature of Hymenomycetes and Ustilaginales.

Heinrich Anton de Bary (1831-1888)

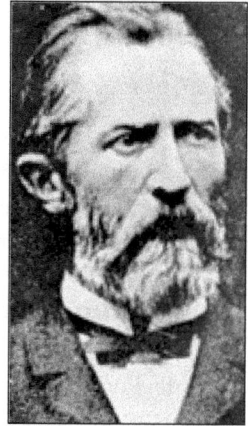

Figure 11: Anton de Bary.

Born in Frankfurt, Germany he was trained in medicine but became botanist. He laid foundations for experimental Plant pathology at 22 years of age. He confirmed findings of Prevost. He studied 'life history of mycetozoa' in 1859; investigated into the 'etiology of late blight of potato' in 1861; proved *Botrytis infestans* as cause; changed the name *Botrytis* to *Phytophthora infestans*; studied the morphology and physiology of parasitism, sexuality of fungi studied rusts, smuts, downy mildew, rots; studied 'heterocious nature of black stem rust of wheat and barley' in 1865; studied damping off (*Pythium sp.*) and vegetable rot *Sclerotinia sclerotiorum*. Studied life cycle of Downy mildew fungi, suggested role of enzymes in host-pathogen interaction.

He wrote several books *viz.*,

✰ 1853 'Unterschungen uber die brand pilze' at 22 years of age.

✰ 1859 'Die mycetozoan'.

✰ 1866 'Morphology and physiology of fungi, lichens and myxomycetes'.

✰ 1884 'Comparative morphology and biology of Fungi, Mycetozoa and Bacteria' -first book on mycology.

✰ He was considered as 'Founder and Father of Modern Plant Pathology' and trained a number of students of whom more than 60 became prominent.

✰ The most noted ones were Oscar Brefeld of Germany; P.A. Millardet of France; M.S. Woronin of USSR; Marshal Ward of UK and Farlow of USA.

1. **Oscar Brefeld (Germany, 1839-1925)** developed pure culture techniques of isolation of plant pathogens and studied life history of cereal smuts.

2. **P. A. Millardet (France, 1838-1902)** discovered Bordeaux mixture for control of downy mildew of grapevine (*Plasmopara viticola*) in1885.

3. **M. S. Woronin (USSR, 1838-1903)** studied the 'Life cycle of club root of cabbage caused by *Plasmodiophora brassicae*'.

4. **Marshal Ward (UK, 1854-1906)** studied on Epidemiology of coffee rust fungus, *Hemileia vastatrix*.

5. **Farlow** studied parasitic fungi and established Farlow Crytogamic Herbarium.

Robert Koch (Germany, 1843-1910)

He enunciated certain criteria or rules to confirm the association of an organism with a disease. These are known as Koch's postulates and are essential even today to prove the microbial etiology or biotic nature of any disease whether in animals or in plants.

The postulates are:

1. The specific organism in question should always be associated with the disease.

2. The organism must be isolated in pure culture and identified.

3. The organism on inoculation to the susceptible plant should produce identical disease symptoms.

4. The organism should be re-isolated from the artificially inoculated plant in pure culture and its identity established.

Edwin John Butler (British mycologist, 1874-1943)

(Stayed in India 1901-1920.) He worked at Imperial Agricultural Research Institute, Pusa (Bihar) for more than 15 years from 1905 to 1919. He was the Founder and first director of Imperial Mycological Institute, Kew (1920-35). He published a Monograph on Pythiaceous and allied fungi. His books a) Fungi and Disease in Plants (1918); b) Fungi of India (with B.R. Bisby) and c) Plant Pathology (with S.G. Jones) (1949). He is considered as the Father of Modern Plant Pathology in India and Father of Indian Mycology.

☆ 1903. Report on 'Spike' disease among sandalwood trees.

☆ 1906. (With J. M. Hayman and W. H. Moreland) Indian wheat rusts. *Mem. Dep. Agric. India, Bot. Ser.* (2) 1, 58 pp. 1 graph, 5 pls. (4 col.).

☆ 1908. Report on coconut palm disease in Travancore. *Bull. Agric. Res. Inst. Pusa*, no. 9, 23 pp.

☆ 1909. *Fomes lucidus* (Leys) Fr. a suspected parasite. *Indian Forester*, 35, 514-518, 1 col. pl.

☆ 1918. Fungi and disease in plants. Thacker, Spink and Co. Calcutta. vi+547 pp. 206 figs.

☆ 1924. Bud-rot of coconut and other palms. *Rep. Imp. Bot. Conf.* Lond. July 1924, 145-147.

☆ 1925. Meteorological conditions and plant diseases. *Int. Ree. Sci. Pract. Agric.* n.s. (2) 3, 369-384.

☆ 1926. The wilt diseases of cotton and sesamum in India. *Agric. J. India*, (4) 21, 268-273, 1pl.

☆ 1931. (With G. R. Bisby) The fungi of India. *Scientific Monograph Imperial Council of Agric. Research* no. 1, xviii+237 pp. 1 map.

☆ 1949. (with S.G. Jones) Plant Pathology. (London: Macmillan and Co., 1949).

E.C. Stakman

From University of Minnasota studied variability of Rust fungi in detail.

B.B. Mundkur

He worked on the control of cotton wilt caused by *Fusarium oxysporum pv.vascatoria* through the varietal resistance. He started Indian Phytopathological Society in 1948 with its journal '*Indian Phytopathology*'. He wrote a text book – "Fungi and Plant diseases". He was responsible for identification and classification of a large number of smut fungi.

K.C. Mehta

He worked on annual recurrence of rusts on wheat, identified no role of barbery in perpetuation of wheat rust in India.

J.F. Dastur (1886-1971)

He was a colleague of E.J. Butler and first Indian born Plant Pathologist studied on diseases of late blight of potato, cotton wilt, diseases of chilli, cotton, foot rot of betelvine, citrus pink disease, studied *Phytophthora* diseases of castor and potato internationally known estd. Pathogen *Phytophthora parasitica* on castor, organised teaching of plant pathology started Agra University, Govt. Agricultural College, Kanpur in 1945. Founder member, Indian Phytopathological Society Fellow, National Institute of Science of India.

T.J. Burril (1839-1916), University of Illinois, USA

First time proved and established etiology of plant disease caused by bacteria '*Eerwinia amylovora*' fire blight of apple and pears -1878.

T.S. Sadasivan

Director, University Botany Laboratory, Madras known for his active school at Madras University worked on fungal wilts, concepts of fusarial toxin, antibiotics in soil and rhizosphere, changes in physiology of host recipient of Birbal Sahni Medal, Shanti Swarup Bhatnagar Awards – 1962, Fellow of Indian Economy of Sciences, Indian Botanical Society and National Institute of Sciences.

Member- Leopoldina Academy of Natural Sciences of Germany.

Editor- Indian Phytopathology, Journal of Indian Botanical Society, Journal of Madras University, Phytopathologische zeitschrift.

Erwin Frink Smith (USA, 1854-1927)

He worked at U.S.D.A. (Illinois) and took an active part in plant Bacterial Research for about 14 years. He started the study of plant bacterial diseases from 1890 onwards and Bacterial wilt of cucurbits in (1893), he published a detailed report of this disease in 1895, Bacterial wilt of Solanaceous crops in 1896 and Black rot of Crucifers in 1987. He was elected as the President of the Society of American Bacterologists in 1906. He wrote the book "Bacteria in relation to plant diseases" in

3 volumes (1905-1914) and "Bacterial diseases of Plants" in 1920. He is considered as "Father of Phytobacteriology".

M.K. Patel

Pioneer in phytobacteriology in India. Established a school of bacteriology at College of Agriculture, Pune and conducted elaborate studies on cultural, morphological biochemical, pathological characteristics of several bacterial plant pathogens, systemic studies in plant bacteriology at College of Agriculture, Pune in 1948. He described new species *Xanthomonas uppalii* on *Ipomoea muricata*. He also reported more than 40 new species of plant pathogenic bacteria belonging to genus *Xanthomonas* (1899-1967) and studied seed transmission of *Xanthomonas campestris* p.v. *malvacearum* causing black arm disease in cotton and suggested hot water treatment at 122°F for 30 min. to control seed borne infection of X. *c. malvacearum*. Suggested the introduction of Family Phytobacteriaceae to include all plant pathogenic bacteria and introduced the post of 'Plant Bacteriologist' at IARI, 1955.

Adolf Eduard Mayer (Germany, 1843-1942)

He started his work in 1880 on mysterious disease in tobacco and published his report in 1886. He called the symptom as 'Mosaik Krankheiten' (Mosaic disease). He showed that this symptom can be transferred through injection of plant sap obtained from affected plant into a healthy plant and conducted the same transmission but after boiling the sap and no disease was produced. So he speculated that a small bacterium or soluble enzyme or toxin is involved in the disease.

Ivanowski (Russia, 1898)

He worked on the mosaic disease of tobacco in Crimea Region of U.S.S.R. He confirmed the report of Mayer that the disease could be transmitted through sap. He showed that sap obtained from infected plant retains its infectivity even after passing through Chamberland filters, which does not allow bacteria to pass through them. So he concluded that the agent is not bacteria but a small bacterium, which he called 'filterable agent'.

Beijerinck (Dutch, 1896)

He made detailed study of tobacco mosaic disease and he reproduced the disease by using sap passed through porcelain filters and found that the sap still retained the infectivity. He experimentally demonstrated that the filterable, infective principle was also diffusible like liquid, later he referred the agent as *'virus'*. He is considered as "**Father of Plant Virology**".

Wendell M. STANLEY (U.S.A., 1935)

He isolated a proteinaceous, crystalline substance from the mosaic affected tobacco plants but could not recognize the nucleoprotein nature in spite of that this was beginning of biochemical era in plant virology. Even after repeated crystallization, the protein was infective. He considered it as globulate protein. So he isolated, crystallized tobacco mosaic virus (TMV) and claimed that viruses were made exclusively of proteins. He was later awarded Nobel Prize for his work.

F.C. Bawden and M.W. Pirie (England, 1936)

They purified the TMV and characterized it chemically as nucleoprotein (Viruses consist of protein and nucleic acid) and observed that TMV contains 95 per cent protein, 5 per cent nucleic acid (RNA). They established that viruses were nucleoproteins.

Mausche, Pfankuch and Ruska (Germany, 1939)

They observed the particles of TMV under the newly constructed Transmission Electron Microscope, and concluded that they were rod-shaped, measuring about 300 x 18 nm.

Doi, Y. *et al.*, and Ishie *et al.* (Japan, 1967)

These two groups of Japanese scientists were the first to identify the mycoplasma like organisms (now called phytoplasmas) in phloem vessels of plants affected by Aster yellows, mulberry dwarf and potato witches' broom and report that the mulberry dwarf can be controlled by with Tetracycline antibiotics.

M.J. Tirumalachar (India)

He worked as the Director of Hindustan Antibiotics Limited, Pimpri, Pune. He conducted exhaustive investigation on smuts and the rusts in India. First time he successfully introduced the use of antibiotics in plant disease management (aureofungin and streptocyclin). He wrote a book 'Ustilagenales' in India (1918) and 'Uredinales' in the world.

C.V. Subramanian (India)

He worked at Botany Laboratory in Madras University. First time he used Sanskrit words to the newly established fungal genera. He wrote a monograph – Hyphomycetes (1971) and a book Hyphomycetes: Taxonomy and Biology (1978).

Raychaudhuri S.P. *et al.* (India)

They reported the control of sandal spike phytoplasma disease with tetracycline (ledermycin and terramycin) and Benlate in 1972.

Howard Taylor Ricketts (1871-1910)

American pathologist after whom the Family Rickettsiaceae and the Order Rickettsiales are named. For the first time a disease associated with Rickettsia was discovered. First observation of fastidious vascular bacteria was reported in 1972.

3

Classification of Plant Diseases

Diseases may be classified in various ways on the basis of:

A. Based on cause;

B. Based on occurrence; and

C. Based on symptoms.

A. Based on Cause

On the basis of cause, the plant diseases are classified into two categories *viz.*, Parasitic and Non-Parasitic.

a. Parasitic Diseases

These are the diseases incited by biotic factors, *i.e.*, other living organisms under a set of suitable environmental conditions. Association of a specific pathogen is essential with these diseases. These diseases are always infectious, sometimes contagious and are transmitted from diseased to healthy plants in the field and from one place to another through various agencies.

Examples

☆ Fungi: Downy mildew of Grapevine – *Plasmopara viticola*

☆ Bacteria: Citrus Canker – *Xanthomonas campestris* pv. *citri*

☆ Viruses: Bhendi Yellow Vein Disease - Bhendi Yellow Vein *begomovirus*

☆ Viroids: Potato spindle tuber - Potato spindle tuber viroid

☆ Fastidious vascular bacteria (RLO's): Citrus greening – *Liberobacter asiaticus*

☆ Phytoplasma: Brinjal little leaf – *Brinjal Little Leaf Phytoplasma*

☆ Spiroplasmas: Citrus stubborn - *Spiroplasma citri*

☆ Protozoa: Hart-rot and sudden wilt of coconut – *Phytomonas* spp.

☆ Algae: Red rust on mango- *Cephaleuros parasiticus*

☆ Parasitic higher plants (phanerogams): Dodder - *Cuscuta* spp.

b. Non-parasitic Diseases

These are the diseases with which no parasite is associated; hence they are called as non-parasitic or abiotic diseases. They remain non-infectious and cannot be transmitted from one diseased plant to another healthy plant. These non-parasitic, non-infectious diseases are due to disturbances in the plant body caused by lack of proper environmental conditions like suitable soil, air, temperatures, oxygen, moisture, pH, atmosphere etc., are the major causes of non-parasitic diseases.

Examples

☆ Low temperature: Potato tuber injury

☆ High temperature: Blossom end rot of citrus fruit

☆ Effect of light: Bean scald

☆ Excessive moisture: Blossom end rot of tomato

☆ Low oxygen: Black heart of potato

☆ Air pollution: Ozone injury to onion, tomato and cucumber.

☆ Chemical injury: Ammonia on apple

☆ Herbicide injury: 2, 4-D on dicot leaf

☆ Nutrient deficiency: Zn on citrus causes 'mottle leaf of citrus' and

☆ Nutrient excess: Internal bark necrosis of Red delicious apple due to excess Manganese.

B. Based on Occurrence

Parasitic diseases are often classified according to their occurrence as epidemic, endemic, sporadic and pandemic diseases.

a. Epidemic/Epiphytotic

The term epidemic is derived from Greek word ("epi-" = "*upon*"; + "demos" = "*people* or *population*" = "epidemos" = "*upon the population*") meaning "among the people" and in true sense applies to those diseases of human beings which appear very virulently among a large section of population. To carry the same sense in the case of plant diseases, the term epiphytotic has been coined. An epiphytotic disease is the one which occurs widely but periodically. It may be present constantly in the locality but assumes severe proportions only on occasions. This is because the environmental conditions favour rapid development of the disease periodically. Thus, environmental factors are the major determining factors.

☆ Ex: Downy mildew of Grapevine – *Plasmopara viticola*

b. Endemic

The word endemic is also derived from Greek (en-= *in*; + dēmos= *people*) meaning "prevalent in and confined to a particular country or district" and is applied to disease. These diseases are natural to one country or part of the earth. When a disease is more or less constantly present from year to year in a moderate to severe form, in a particular country or part of the earth, it is called as endemic disease to that area.

   ☆ Ex: Club root of cabbage - *Plasmodiophora brassicae.*

   ☆ Wart disease of potato - *Synchitrium endobioticum.*

c. Sporadic

Sporadic disease is the one which occurs at very irregular intervals and locations and in relatively few instances.

   ☆ Ex: Angular leaf spot of cucumber - *Pseudomonas lachrymans.*

d. Pandemic

These occur all over the world across the continents and result in mass mortality of people.

   ☆ Ex: Late blight of potato - *Phytophthora infestans.*

C. Based on Symptoms

Based on symptom, diseases are classified into 3 types.

   a) Necrotic disease

   b) Hyperplastic/Hypertrophic disease

   c) Hypoplastic/Hypotrophic disease

a. Necrotic Diseases

The diseases that involve the death of the tissue due to the derangement of cells are termed as Necrotic diseases. Necrotic diseases involve decay or rotting.

The different necrotic diseases are:

   i) Wilts: They are characterized by destruction or necrosis of vascular tissue resulting in dying of entire plant. The plants suffer from dehydration and show the symptoms of drought.

   Ex: Panama Wilt of banana - *Fusarium oxysporium* f.sp. *cubense.*

   ii) Spots: The spots are self-limiting necrotic areas or the necrosis is local on leaf lamina, stem or fruit.

   Ex: Chillies anthracnose - *Collectotrichum caspcii.*

   iii) Blights: Blights are characterized by rapid and extensive necrosis *i.e.,* quick death of cells, tissues or whole plant or plant parts.

Ex: Late blight of potato - *Phytopthora infestans*.

iv) ***Rots***: They are characterized by necrosis of parenchyma, collenchyma and pith tissues in which the necrosis is not localized.

Ex: Bud rot of palms - *Phytopthora palmivora*

Soft rot of vegetable - *Erwinia caratovora*

v) ***Damping Off***: Necrosis of basal portion of stem or crown region of seedlings, resulting in toppling down of seedlings or death of seedlings in groups.

Ex: Damping off of solanaceous plants - *Pythium aphanidermatum*.

vi) ***Canker***: This canker is due to necrosis of woody tissue in which the infection is deep-seated and hypertrophy of cambium tissues.

Ex: Citrus canker - *Xanthomonas campestris* pv. *Citrus*

Guava fruit canker - *Pestalotia psidi*.

vii) ***Scab***: It is also a necrosis which is superficial and restricted to epidermal region.

Ex: Citrus scab *Elsinoe fawcettii*

Apple scab *Venturia inequalis*.

b. Hyperplastic/Hypertrophic Diseases

They are characterized by over-growth of the tissue due to either hyperplasia or hypertrophy.

☆ *Hyperplasia*: It is increase in number of cells due to excess cell division.

Ex: Crown gall of apple and pears - *Agrobacterium tumefaciens*

Club root of cabbage – *Plasmodiophora brassicae*

☆ *Hypertrophy*: It is abnormal increase in size of cells.

Ex: Tumors: Wound tumor of clover – Wound tumor virus.

Wart: Wart of potato – *Synchitrium endobiotium*.

Galls: Stem gall of coriander - *Protomyces macrosporus*.

Woody gall: Woody gall of citrus – Viral disease.

Blisters: White rust of crucifers – *Albugo candida*.

White pine blister rust – *Cronartium ribicola*.

Witches' brooms: Potato witches' broom – Phytoplasma.

c. Hypoplastic/Hypotrophic Diseases

They are characterized by under-development of tissues or stunting or dwarfing of plant due to hypoplasty or hypotrophy.

☆ *Hypoplasia* – Decrease in normal growth of the tissue due to reduced cell division.

Ex: Citrus Tristeza disease – Citrus Tristeza *closterovirus*

Chrysanthemum stunt – Chrysanthemum stunt viroid.

☆ *Hypotrophy* - Decrease in normal growth of the tissue due to reduced cell size.

Ex: Aster yellows – *Phytoplasma*

Downy mildew of Grapevine – *Plasmopara viticola.*

4

Terms and Concepts Used in Plant Pathology

Disease and Disorder

These two terms carry the same meaning *i.e.*, malfunctioning of physiological processes in the plant. However, if the malfunctioning of the plant is due to biotic cause (living organism) which is infectious, it is termed as disease, while the malfunctioning due to abiotic (non-living) cause which is non- infectious, it is termed disorder.

Causal Organism/Causal Agent

It is an organism which is a part of causal complex to cause a disease. Most causal organisms are parasitic.

Ex: *Plasmopara viticola*- causal organism of downy mildew of grapes.

Pathogen

It is an entity, usually a micro-organism that can incite a disease.

Parasite

It is an organism living on or in another living organism (host) and obtaining food from the latter.

Pathogenicity

The ability of a pathogen to cause a disease.

Pathogenesis

The sequence of events in disease development from initial contact between pathogen and host to completion of syndrome.

Disease Cycle

The sequence of events in recurrence of a disease in successive seasons.

Symptom

The external and internal reactions or alterations expressed by a plant externally as a result of a disease.

Ex: Sigatoka disease of banana – *Mycosphaerella musicale*.

Sign

The visible structure of a pathogen or its parts or products seen on diseased host tissue.

Ex: Powdery mass of powdery mildew fungi – *Eryciphales* order.

Pycnidia in leaf spots caused by *Septoria lycopersici* on tomato.

Syndrome

The totality of effects produced in a plant by a disease. This includes both symptoms and signs.

Biotroph

An organism which, regardless of ease with which they can be cultured in nature, obtains its food from the living tissues on which it completes life cycle (or) an organism that can live and multiply only on another living organism.

Ex: *Plasmopara viticola* – Downy mildew of Grapevine.

Hemibiotroph

An organism which attacks living tissues in the same way as biotrophs, but will continue to grow and reproduce even after tissue is dead.

Ex: *Alternaria solani* – Early blight of potato and tomato.

Perthotroph

An organism which kills host tissue in advance of penetration and then lives saprophytically.

Ex: *Fusarium oxysporum* f. sp. *cubense* – Panama Wilt of Banana.

Necrotroph

An organism which has no relation with living cells and obtains its food from dead organic tissues.

Ex. *Rhizopus*.

Inoculum

The pathogen or its parts that can cause infection on the host.

Inoculum Potential

It is defined as the number of independent infections that are likely to occur in a given situation in a population of susceptible healthy tissues. This is considered to be the resultant action of the environment, the virulence of the pathogen to establish an infection, the susceptibility of the host and the amount of inoculum used.

Infection

The establishment of a parasite within a host plant.

Incubation Period

The period of time between penetration of a host by a pathogen and the first appearance of symptoms on the host.

Predisposition

It is the condition of the host which operates before infection by a pathogen and its affect on the susceptibility of the host rather than directly affecting the pathogen.

Hypersensitivity

Increased sensitivity by the host at the site of infection as shown by rapid cell death which prevents further growth of the pathogen and spread of infection.

Disease Triangle

There are three factors for the development of a disease *viz.*, virulent pathogen, susceptible host and favorable environment for the pathogen.

The interaction of host, pathogen and environment have often visualised as a triangle, generally referred to as disease triangle. Each side of the triangle represents one of the three components. The size of each side is proportional to the sum total of the characteristics of each component that favour the disease. If the three components of the disease could be quantified, the area of triangle would represent the amount of disease in a plant.

Disease Pyramid/Tetrahedron

The disease triangle, used to describe interaction of three components of plant disease, can be expanded by including time as the fourth component. The amount of each of the three components of the triangle as well as their effect on each other in the development of disease is affected by time (*e.g.* the duration of favorable weather conditions at which the host and the pathogen may co-exist). The interaction of these four components can be visualised as a tetrahedron or a pyramid, in which each plane represents one of the components. The figure is referred to as disease pyramid or tetrahedron. If the four components of the disease pyramid could be quantified, the volume of tetrahedron would be proportional to the amount of disease on a plant or in a plant population.

5

Classification of Fungi

Numerous schemes of classification have been proposed and some have been adopted. A generally accepted scheme for fungal classification has been published by the Commonwealth Mycological Institute (1983) and is reproduced here. The scheme is based on common ending for order, class, divisions, names etc. These are Division: -mycota; Sub-division: -mycotina; Class: -mycetes; Sub-class: -mycetidae; Order: -ales; and Family-ceae.

Kingdom:	Mycota	
Division:	1. Myxomycota	2. Eumycota
	↓	↓
	Class	Sub-Divisions
	↓	↓
	Plasmodiophoromycetes	1. Mastigomycotina
		2. Zygomycotina
		3. Ascomycotina
		4. Basidiomycotina
		5. Deutermycotina

Important Characters

Division 1: Myxomycota

☆ Slime moulds

☆ Plasmodial forms

☆ Thallus is plasmodium

☆ True mycelium is absent.

Class I: Plasmodiophoromycetes

☆ Endoparasitic slime moulds.

☆ Obligate parasites of vascular plants

☆ Thallus is plasmodium

    a) Sporangiogenous Plasmodium - Sporangial zoospores

    b) Cystogenous plasmodium – Cyst Zoospores

☆ Biflagellate Zoospores – Heterocont zoospores.

☆ Sexual reproduction – Isogamous planogametic copulation.

☆ Cause hypertrophy and hyperplasia of host tissue.

Division 2: Eumycota

☆ True fungi.

☆ Non-plasmodial filamentous forms with cell wall.

☆ Well-developed filamentous thallus.

Sub-Division

a) *Mastigomycotina*

☆ Motile spores (Zoospores) are present.

☆ Flagellate zoospores

☆ Sexual spores – Oospore

☆ Sexual reproduction - gametangial contact (or) gametangial copulation

b) *Zygomycotina*

☆ No motile spores.

☆ Produce non-motile spores – Aplanospores

☆ Well-developed coenocytic mycelium

☆ Sexual reproduction – gametangial copulation

c) *Ascomycotina*

☆ They are called 'sac fungi'.

☆ No motile spores

☆ Fruiting body – Ascus (Ascocarp)

☆ Sexual spore – Ascospore

☆ Asexual spore – Conidia

☆ Well-developed septate mycelium

☆ Presence of brief dikaryotic phase

☆ Sexual reproduction – gametangial contact

d) *Basidiomycotina*

☆ The members of basidiomycotina are called club fungi as the basidium is club-shaped

☆ Septate mycelium usually with binucleate cell

☆ Presence of dolipore septum

☆ No motile spores

☆ Fruiting body – Basidiocarp

☆ Sexual spore – Basidiospores

☆ Asexual spores – Conidia

☆ Dikaryotic phase dominates the life cycle

☆ Presence of clamp connections

e) *Deuteromycotina*

☆ Fungi imperfecti (Technical name)

☆ Imperfect fungi (common name)

☆ Well-developed septate mycelium

☆ No motile spores

☆ No sexual spores

☆ Produce only asexual spores called conidia

☆ Perfect stages have been found in sub-divisions, Ascomycotina and Basidiomycotina.

Key to Each Sub-division with Examples and Life Cycles of Representative Members

Division: Myxomycota

Class: Plasmodiophoromycetes

General Characters

1. These are obligate endoparasites consisting of a naked plasmodial thallus.

2. The plasmodial thallus is of two types

   (a) Cystogenous plasmodium and (b) Sporangiogenous plasmodium.

3. Zoospores are biflagellate with two anteriorly or laterally whip lash flagella of unequal size (Arisokont).

4. The genera cause abnormal elongation of cells (hypertrophy) and cell division (hyperplasia).

5. Nuclear division by pro-mitosis or cruciform division.

6. This class includes 16 genera; among them *Plasmodiophora*, *Spongospora* and *Polymyxa* are important.

Typical Example of Life Cycles

Life Cycle of *Plasmodiophora brassicae* Causing Club-root of Cabbage

Division: Myxomycota

Class: Plasmodiophoromycetes

Order: Plasmodiophorales

Family: Plasmodiophoraceae

Genus: *Plasmodiophora*

Species: *P. brassicae*

The thallus, known as plasmodium, is characterized by the presence of naked multinucleate motile mass of protoplasm. Most of life cycle is spent in the root cells of host. When the host dies and the roots disintegrate, minute, round, uninucleate, haploid resting spores enveloped in a smooth chitinous wall of the organism are liberated into the soil.

These spores survive in soil for 5 to 8 years under favorable conditions. In the presence of host plant each spore germinates giving rise to a uninucleate bean-

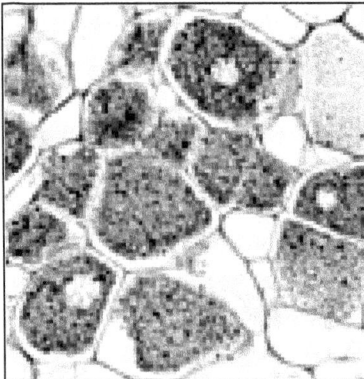

Figure 12: *Plasmodiophora* in Cells.

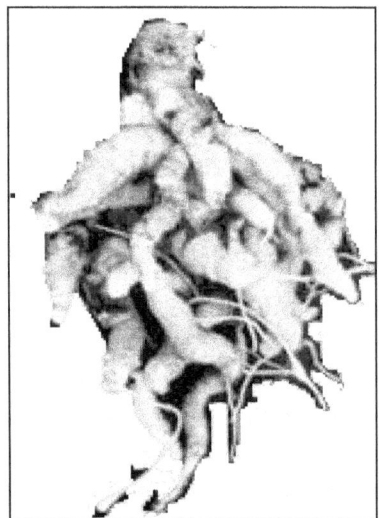

Figure 13: Club-root Symptoms.

shaped biflagellate zoospores (swarm cells). In the absence of host cells, these spores perish. Before infecting the host the zoospore becomes amoeboid. The entire body of amoeba enters the host cell within the root hair or epidermal cells. A small uninucleate stage is seen first. As the amoeba grows, its nucleus divides and transforms into small multinucleate plasmodium. Each nucleus is haploid. Then the plasmodium cleaves into many multinucleate portions (protoplasts). Each protoplast is surrounded by a thin, hyaline wall and develops into gametangia (Zoosporangium). Then the nuclear division takes place in the gametangium which results in the formation 4-8 spindle-shaped planogametes (Zoospores or gametes). They are released from gametangia and fuse in pairs. Plasmogamy and Karyogamy takes place, resulting in the formation of a uninucleate diploid zygote from each pair. The zygote looses its flagella and the parasite is in the form of diploid amoeba. The amoeba further migrates from the root hair into the cortical or other cells and grows into a plasmodium by repeated divisions of zygote nucleus. This further result in hypertrophy and hyperplasia of host cells. This division of host cells is a major factor in the multiplication of the parasite and the entire plasmodium is converted into a mass of globose resting spores each of which is haploid and surrounded by a wall.

The spores are crowded together within the host cells and they are released on the disintegration of the roots and then the life cycle starts again.

Division: Eumycota

Sub-Division-1: MASTIGOMYCOTINA

Members of this group cause most destructive plant diseases like downy mildews, blights, white rusts etc. The soil inhabiting ones cause serious root-rot and collar-rots and also damping off. Others often cause spoilage of various fruits and vegetables either in transit or in storage. Few others are parasites on insects while some others cause human diseases.

Class: OOMYCETES

The fungi which form oospore as sexual spore are called Oomycetes, and type of sexual reproduction characterized by oospore formation is called the 'oomycetous' type. The sexual identity of male and female gametangia is evident *i.e.,* they differ in size and shape, the female being larger-than the male. They also differ in function. The male is very active while the female reproductive organ acts as a passive receptive cell which then matures into oospores. The fertilization tube does not function as a conjugation tube in most cases but pierces oogonial wall and passage of one or more nuclei directly into the oogonium to fertilize it, finally resulting in the thick-walled oospore, lying free in the oogonium.

Life Cycle of *Pythium aphanidermatum* Causing Damping Off of Seedlings

Division: Eumycota

Sub-Division: Mastigomycotina

Class: Oomycetes

Order: Peronosporales

Family: Pythiaceae

Genus: *Pythium*

Species: *P. aphanidermatum*

Pythiaceae: Sporangiophores not sharply differentiated from hyphae. Only a few have differentiated sporangiophores. Sporangia are borne successively.

The fungus is a common soil inhabitant. It is responsible for a number of important crop diseases like "Damping off" of tobacco, chillies, and tomato. It causes other serious diseases like soft-rot of ginger and foot-rot of papaya. The damping off disease is a very common nursery disease. The disease occurs at any stage of the seedling growth but usually manifests itself about two weeks after germination. Affected seedlings become pale green and show brown decaying cortex at ground level. The seedlings collapse and topple over as a result of the weakening of the tissues at the base (crown) of the stem. The disease is favored by excessive soil moisture, high atmospheric humidity and overcrowding of seedlings. The fungus is normally a saprophyte but becomes a parasite under suitable conditions and hence it is a facultative parasite.

The vegetative portion of the fungus is made up of a hyaline branched mycelium and septa are absent. The fungus reproduces by both the methods *viz.*, asexual and sexual means.

Asexual Reproduction

Some of the hyphal branches produce swollen structures called sporangia. They are irregularly lobed and are cut off from the main hyphae by a septum. This structure is full of granular protoplasm. It may be terminal or intercalary. Under favorable conditions of temperature, food supply and sufficient oxygen, the sporangium germinates by giving rise to a tubular outgrowth from one of the lobes. This structure ends in a spherical sac called as vesicle. The protoplasmic content of the sporangium passes into this. After all the protoplasm has moved, the protoplasm divides into a number of separate bits. Each bit develops into a kidney-shaped zoospore with two cilia attached on the concave side. The zoospores are only naked bits of protoplasm without any wall or membrane. Shortly the vesicle bursts open liberating the zoospores. The zoospores swim in water for some time (1/2 hour), shed their flagella and become rounded and finally surround itself with a wall. The zoospore in this condition is called as encysted zoospore. Later on the encysted zoospore germinates producing a tubular outgrowth called germ tube and continues to grow further and develops into a new mycelium.

Sexual Reproduction

At the end of certain hyphal threads, specialized structures are produced. They are also produced rarely intercalary. They are cut off from the main hyphae by septa. These are called oogonia representing the female sexual organ and antheridium representing the male sexual organ. The oogonia have thin colourless walls to begin with, later turning into pale yellow. In the beginning the oogonium is

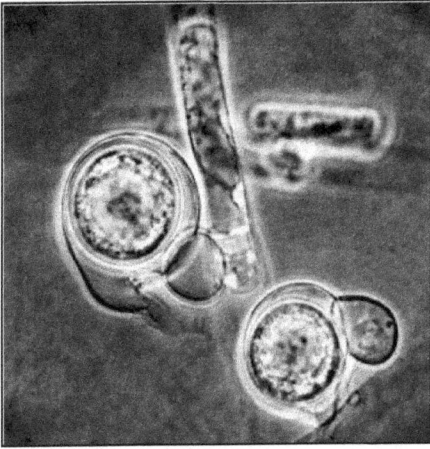

Figure 14: *Pythium*-Antheridium and Oogonium.

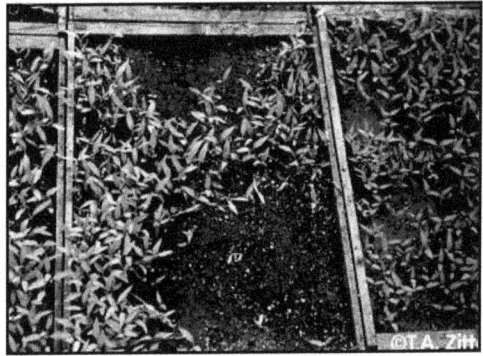

Figure 15: Damping Off.

filled with granular protoplasm but at maturity the protoplasm gets differentiated into a dense central region called oosphere and a clear peripheral layer. Hyphal branches bearing a cylindrical or club-shaped structure called antheridium may arise anywhere along the oogonial stalk (monoclinous) or from another branch of the thallus (diclinous). The antheridium is cut off from the hypha by a septum. The antheridium may be terminal or intercalary. It may arise either from the same mycelium. The organs are brought together by the curvature of the hyphae so that the tip of the antheridium is described as farraginous (as against amphigynous). At the point of contact the wall between them gets dissolved and a small projection or fertilization tube arising from the antheridium penetrates into the oosphere. The contents of the antheridium flow in and thus the mixing of the protoplasmic contents of oosphere and antheridium is effected. This is subsequently followed with the thick wall formed around the fertilized oosphere and the structure with the thick wall is called oospore. The oospore wall is yellowish brown in colour. The oospore does not fill the cavity of the oogonium completely (aplerotic). The wall of the oogonium is persistent.

The oospores can resist adverse conditions. After a period of rest, under favorable conditions, the oospores germinate by producing a germ tube which branches and gives rise to mycelium.

Life Cycle of *Phytophthora infestans* Causing Late Blight of Potato

Division: Eumycota

Sub-Division: Mastigomycotina

Class: Oomycetes

Order: Peronosporales

Family: Pythiaceae

Genus: *Phytophthora*

Species: *P. infestans*

The genus *Phytophthora* is closely allied to Pythium. It contains many destructive plant pathogens hence is very important. The following are some of the important diseases caused by *Phytophthora* species.

1. *P. palmivora*: Leaf fall and fruit-rot of citrus, But-rot of coconut
2. *P. colocasiae:* Blight disease on colocasia
3. *P. infestans*: Late-blight of potato
4. *P. meadii:* Leaf fall of rubber
5. *P. arecae:* Mahali or Koleroga of arecanut.

Phytophthora infestans causes a serious disease on potato, commonly called late blight disease. It first appears as circular or irregular water-soaked spots, usually at the tips or edges of the lower leaves. In moist weather, the spots enlarge rapidly and form brown, blighted areas with indefinite borders, although frequently a pale yellowish green zone surrounds the rapidly expending lesions. A zone of white, downy fungus growth appears at the border of the lesions on the undersides of the leaves. Soon the entire leaflet and then all the leaflets on a leaf are infected, die, and become limp. Under continuous wet conditions, all tender parts above ground get blighted and quickly rot away, giving a characteristic odour. The fungus infects tubers which show shallow, more or less irregular, purplish black dry rot. When opened, the affected tissue appears water-soaked, dark, some-what reddish brown, and extending up to 5-15 mm deep into the flesh of the tuber. Later, tuber may rot in association with soft-rot bacteria giving a putrid, offensive odour.

The vegetative portion of mycelium consists of much branched hyaline hyphae which are aseptate, intercellular (*i.e.,* between the host cells) and are provided with long, slender, unbranched haustoria for absorbing nourishment from the host. After growing sufficiently inside the host, the fungus begins to reproduce both asexually and sexually.

Asexual Reproduction

Under suitable conditions of temperature and moisture, certain specialized structures called sporangiophores are produced on the surface of the leaves. Pear-shaped sporangia develop singly at the tips. The sporangia are hyaline and full of granular protoplasm. They are attached to the sporangiophores at the broader base. The walls of sporangia at the narrow end are slightly thicker and bear beak-like structures called papilla. The sporangia germinate either directly by producing germ tubes or indirectly by producing zoospores. Many zoospores which are uniform and biflagellate may be formed within the sporangium. They are released by the rupture of the papilla. The zoospores swim about for sometime, shed their cilia, come to rest, and encyst. Under favorable conditions they germinate by producing germ tubes. This type of germination of the sporangium (*i.e.,* production of zoospores) is called indirect method of germination. Under certain other conditions (warmer)

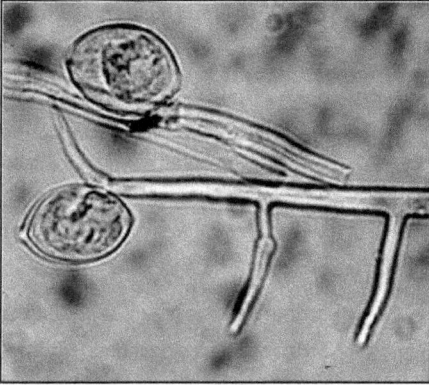

Figure 16: Sporangiophore and Sporangia of *Phytophthora*.

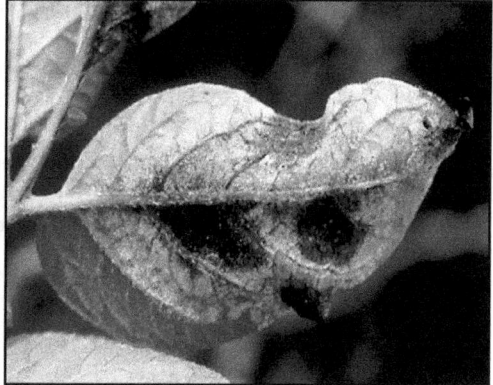

Figure 17: Late Blight of Potato.

the sporangia germinate directly producing the germ tube instead of zoospore. This is called direct method of germination. The method of germination is largely governed by temperature. Low temperature favours zoospore production.

Sexual Reproduction

The sexual organs *viz.*, oogonium and antheridium are produced separately. The antheridium is first developed. The oogonium perforates the wall of antheridium and penetrates into it finally emerging out at the other side as spherical structures. While passing through the antheridium, fertilization is effected. A single male nucleus enters the oogonium. Inside the spherical structure, a thick-walled oospore develops.

The oospores are smooth, spherical, thick-walled and lie free in the oogonium. They do not completely fill the oogonial cavity and the oospore germinates by a germ tube which develops into mycelium.

Heterothallism: Some isolates of *Phytophthora* sp. *e.g.*, *P. palmivora* do not produce oospores in nature. The different thalli of opposite sex potentialities are essential to bring about sexual reproduction. There is no morphological difference between the two thalli but they differ in their physiological characters. Only when they are brought together and the contact is affected that the oopores are formed. In such cases one of the thalli is called positive (plus) and the other negative (minus). It is only when the plus and minus isolates are brought together that sexual spores are produced. Such a phenomenon is called heterothallism and the species exhibiting the phenomenon are called heterothallic species.

Ex: *P. palmivora* and *P. arecae*. *Phytophthora* spp. are facultative saprophytes *i.e.*, they are normally parasites but sometimes exhibit saprophytic habits.

The chief distinction between the genera *Pythium* and *Phytophthora* is in the mode of sporangial germination. In general, no vesicle is formed in *Phytophthora*.

Differences between *Pythium* and *Phytophthora*

Character	Pythium	Phytophthora
1. Mycelium	Inter and Intracellular. No haustoria. Homothallic	Intercellular with haustoria. Both homothallic and heterothallic
2. Sporangiophore	Indistinct from hyphae. Determinate growth	Distinct with nodal swelling. Indeterminate growth
3. Sporangia	Globose/loabed/terminal/intercalary. Papillum not procont	Lemon-shaped and terminal. Papillum present
4. Zoospores	Differentiated in a vesicle	No vesicle is formed. Differentiate in sporangia and migrate to vesicle.
5. Antheridium	Paragynous	Perigynous/Amphigynous
6. Thallus	Homothallic	Heterothallic
7. Asexual reproduction	Zoospores in sporangia	Zoospores is sporangia and chlamydospores
8. Oospores	Aplenetic	Aplenetic
9. Appressorium	Not formed	Formed
10. Oogonial wall	Hyaline, spiny	Brown, warty

Life Cycle of *Plasmopara viticola* Causing Downy Mildew of Grapes

Division: Eumycota

Sub-Division: Mastigomycotina

Class: Oomycetes

Order: Peronosporales

Family: Peronosporaceae

Genus: *Plasmopara*

Species: *P. viticola*

The family Peronosporaceae consists of 17 genera, comprising more than 600 species. Most of them are called 'downy mildews'. The closest relative of Peronosporaceae is *Phytophthora*.

Peronosporaceae are obligate, biotrophic plant pathogens. They parasitize their host plants as an intercellular mycelium using haustoria to penetrate the host cells. The downy mildews reproduce asexually by releasing sporangia or conidia. These may collectively be referred to as Conidiosporangia. Sexual reproduction is via oospores.

Parasitized plants are angiosperms, most Peronosporaceae are pathogens of dicots. Some downy mildew genera have a more restricted host range, *e.g.* Basidiophora, Paraperonospora, Protobremia and Bremia on Asteraceae; Perofascia and Hyaloperonospora almost only on Brassicaceae; Viennotia, Graminivora, Poakatesthia, Sclerospora and Peronosclerospora on Poaceae, Plasmoverna on Ranunculaceae. The largest genera, Peronospora and Plasmopara, have a very wide host range.

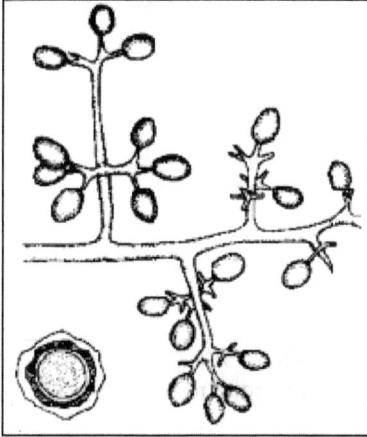

Figure 18: Sporangiophore,   **Figure 19: Downy Mildew on Grapevine.**
Sporangia and Oospore of
P. viticola.

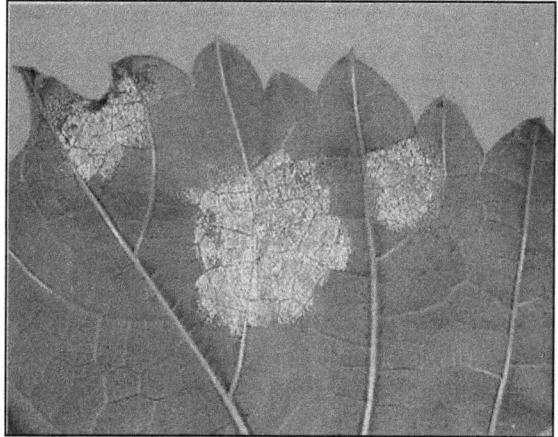

Peronosporaceae of economic importance include *Plasmopara viticola* on grapevines, *Peronospora tabacina* on tobacco, *Bremia lactucae* on lettuce, *Plasmopara halstedii* on sunflower, and *Pseudoperonospora cubensis* on cucumber.

Grapevine downy mildew pathogen, *Plasmopara viticola*, overwinters as oospores chiefly within fallen leaves in and around the vineyard. It also survives as dormant mycelium in infected twigs. In early spring, as soon as temperatures reach 11°C, the oospores germinate in water to form sporangia. Motile zoospores are produced in sporangia and are dispersed onto host grape tissue by rain splash.

Zoospores germinate under optimum conditions (18 to 24°C and free moisture) in less than 90 minutes. They penetrate the lower surface of young leaves, shoots and tendrils through the stomata and spread throughout the tissue. During humid or wet warm weather the fungus produces a white cottony growth of sporangiophores on the bunch rachis or on the lower leaf surface. Sporangia are produced on these sporangiophores followed by production of zoospores in the sporangia. During rainy atmosphere zoospores are released and spread by rain splashes to other host tissues, causing fresh infections. Continued development of downy mildew during the season depends on the frequency of suitable wetting periods and the presence of susceptible host tissue. Late season infections can develop during prolonged heavy dew or fog. At the end of the growing season, sexual spores called 'oospores' are formed by fusion of antheridium and oogonium within diseased leaves. The oospores are the resting spores which over winter on the ground until they germinate the following spring.

Life Cycle of *Albugo candida* Causing White Rust/Blister on Crucifers

Division: Eumycota

Sub-Division: Mastigomycotina

Class: Oomycetes

Order: Peronosporales

Family: Albuginaceae

Genus: *Albugo*

Species: *A. candida*

Albugo is the only genus in the family Albuginaceae

Albugo candida – White rust/blister on Cruciferaceae

Albugo bliti – White rust/blister on Amaranthaceae

All the members of the family cause diseases called "White Rusts". They are called so because of their superficial resemblance to the true rusts incited by Basidiomycotina but white in colour.

All the members of this family are obligate parasites. They attack a wide range of host plants belonging to families Cruciferae (Cabbage, Radish, Turnip, and Mustard), Amaranthaceae, Convolvulaceae, Compesitae etc. All parts of the host plant are affected except roots. The fungus produces white or creamy yellow pustules of varying sizes and shapes and very often they coalesce together forming bigger patches. In case of systemic infections, the pustules develop in concentric rings. They are formed below the epidermis but with the pressure exerted by the outward growth of chains of sporangia, the epidermis is ruptured and a powdery mass appears on the surface of the leaves. The leaves are mainly attacked and the pustules are on the lower surface generally but in severe cases on both sides. In some cases the fungus affects the stem also causing the entire stem to get uniformly swollen, crinkled and deformed. The dormant buds proliferate resulting in a bushy growth of the plant. Affected flowers show various malformations and discolouration. Stamens may be converted into green leafy structures or sometimes into club-shaped sterile structures. Very often the pistils are subjected to hypertrophy and swell into sacs. In some cases, the habit of the plant is altered.

The mycelium is aseptate, coarse and hyaline. It is strictly intercellular and provided with globular or rarely knob-shaped haustoria. It reproduces both asexually and sexually.

Asexual Reproduction

After growing vigorously inside the host, the internal mycelium collects below the epidermis and gives rise to compact, club-shaped, unbranched sporangiophores. Spherical, thin-walled hyaline sporangia are produced at the tips of the sporangiophores in a basipetal chain. The top most sporangium has a thicker wall and is the oldest. However, the first sporangium does not germinate usually. The outward growth of the chain exerts considerable pressure on the epidermis which bursts open exposing the contents of the sorus (sori-pl). The sporangia in the chain are separated from each other by means of gelatinous disjunction discs in between the sporangia called isthmus. When the sorus is exposed the gelatinous disc dries up and the sporangia are blown by winds. Sporangia are normally globose but during their formation flattened sides may form resulting in cubic or polyhedral shapes.

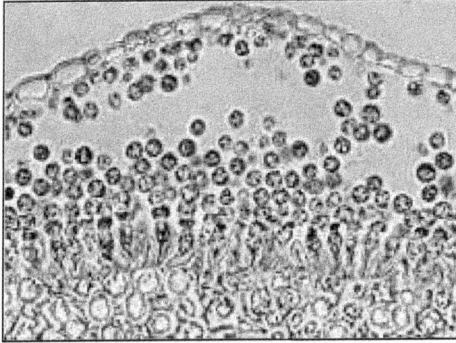

Figure 20: Sporangiophores and Sporangia of *Albugo* spp. in Cross-Section of Leaf Infected with White Rust.

The sporangia are short-lived and easily dry up when exposed. Under favorable conditions of moisture and temperature, they germinate giving rise to biciliate zoospores which are also known as swarm spores. They swim for sometime, come to rest and germinate giving rise to germ tubes.

Sexual Reproduction

Sexuality is well developed in this family and the sexual organs *viz.*, antheridium and oogonium are produced within the host cell. The oogonium is a globose structure and develops from a terminal and intercalary swelling of the hyphae. Its contents are differentiated into denser zone called ooplasm. The antheridium is clavate and applies itself to the side of the oogonium. As soon as they come in contact with each other, the fertilization tube from antheridium enters the oogonium, reaches the ooplasm, ruptures its wall and finally fertilization is effected.

In *A. candida*, a single male nucleus fuses with a single female nucleus. Both antheridium and oogonium are multinucleate at the start but only one nucleus in each finally remains functional.

The oospore develops a thick wall with characteristic markings or thickenings on the outer wall. In case of *A. candida* the oospore wall is of tuberculation type. The oospore is a resting spore. It is liberated by the disintegration of the host tissues. Its germination takes place after a period of rest. Under favorable conditions the outer wall of the oospore bursts open and the inner wall bulges out like a vesicle, and zoospores are extruded into the vesicle in a mass. They are then liberated by the rupture of the vesicle. The zoospores germinate giving rise to mycelium. This family comprises only one genus *viz.*, *Albugo* and the species are separated into two groups' *viz.*, the tuberculate and the reticulate type, based on the character of the markings on the outer wall of the oospores and the host plant involved.

Tuberculate type – *A. ipomea-panduratae* and *A. candida*

Reticulate type – *A. bliti* and *A. portulacae*

Division: Eumycota

Sub-Division-2: ZYGOMYCOTINA

Zygomycotina are characterized by the production of Zygospores. The swarm spores (motile) are completely lacking and the sexual reproduction is zygomycetous. The differentiation of the female and male gametangia is not evident. They are usually morphologically similar and hence not designated as antheridium or oogonium. Direct copulation takes place in all the cases. The walls of the two sexual organs are absorbed and a common wall results in which the two protoplasts are completely merged. In many cases the fusion cell itself gets enlarged and the individuality of copulating gametangia is completely obliterated. The fusion nucleus and protoplasm finally round up, assumes a wall and matures into zygospores. The gametangial wall enveloping the fusion protoplasm becomes greatly thickened and serves as the wall of the spore. Fusion of one or more pairs of nuclei occurs in the zygospore. The functional zygospore corresponds to the oospore is being a resting spore.

This sub-division includes 2 classes.

1. Trichomycetes, and

2. Zygomycetes.

The Class Zygomycetes includes 3 orders a) Entomophthorales b) Zoophagales c) Mucorales.

Entomophthorales: Asexual reproduction chiefly by means of conidia which are violently discharged, mostly entomogenous.

Mucorales: Asexual reproduction chiefly by means of sporangia containing one or more aplanospores.

Main characteristics of the Mucorales:

1. Complete absence of motile cells and consequently of flagella.

2. Sexual reproduction by gametangial copulation between two gametangia which are undifferentiated morphologically and the formation of a zygospore.

Life Cycle of *Rhizopus stolonifer* Causing Soft Rot of Sweet Potato and Mould on Bread

Division: Eumycota

Sub-Division: Zygomycotina

Class: Zygomycetes;

Order: Mucorales;

Family: Mucoraceae;

Genus: *Rhizopus*

Species: *R. stolonifer*

The fungus is a saprophyte or weak parasite. Mycelium is coenocytic but well-developed. Hyphae are of three types:

a) *Rhizoides*: Short hyphae growing in a root-like fashion towards the substratum, useful for anchoring the thallus to the substratum and to absorb nutrients.

b) *Stolons/runners*: Aerial hyphae which grow on the surface of substratum and connect two rhizodal points.

c) *Sporangiophores*: Erect, unbranched, grown vertically, produced in groups opposite to the Rhizoidal points and teminate like a sac like structure called sporangium.

Asexual Reproduction

Sporangia are produced at the tip of sporangiophores. Sporangia are large, globose with many asexual spores known as sporangiospores and a sterile structure called columella.

Sexual Reproduction

This is accomplished by iso-gametangial copulation resulting in production of zygospores which are thick-walled and warty.

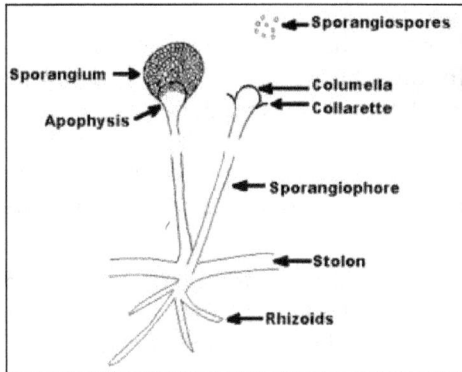

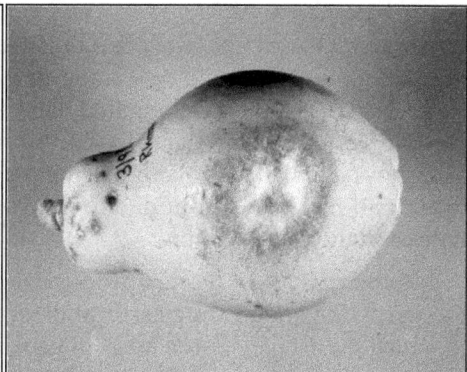

Figure 21: *Rhizopus*.   **Figure 22: *Rhizopus* Fruit-Rot of Papaya.**

Comparison of the Characters of Mastigomycotina and Zygomycotina

Sl.No.	Mastigomycotina	Zygomycotina
1.	Asexual reproduction is by production of motile zoospores (Planospores)	Asexual reproduction is by production of non-motile spores (Aplanospores)
2.	Sexual reproduction results in oospores	Zygospores are sexual spores
3.	There is difference in the size, shape and activities of male and female gametangia	No difference
4.	Male nucleus reaches the egg cell through a fertilization tube	Direct copulation takes place
5.	The cell wall contains cellulose	The cell wall contains chitin

Division: Eumycota

Sub Division-3: ASCOMYCOTINA (The sac fungi)

These are more advanced than the members of Mastigomycotina. The yeasts, the black moulds, the common green moulds, the powdery mildews, the morels and the truffles are among the well known fungi under Ascomycotina. Just as the sporangium is the characteristic structure for the Mastigomycotina, so is the ascus for the Ascomycotina. The ascus is a sac-like structure containing a definite number of ascospores which may vary from one to over a thousand according to the species formed as a result of sexual reproduction. Eight ascospores in each ascus is the typical number.

Sexual reproduction in the Ascomycotina is by the union of two compatible nuclei, which are brought together by Spermatisation or gametangial contact or gametangial conjugation or Somatogamy. The two nuclei do not fuse soon but form a functional pair and undergo conjugate division resulting in a number of dikaryotic cells. Nuclear fusion takes place in the ascus mother-cell which develops into the ascus. Then meiosis of the diploid nucleus in the zygote occurs and four haploid nuclei are produced which divide once more mitotically and form eight nuclei which go to form eight ascospores in the ascus.

Asci and Ascospores

In many cases, the asci are elongated or club-shaped or cylindrical. In some, they are globose or ovoid or rectangular. In some the asci are septate. Asci may be stalked or sessile. Sterile elongated hairs arise between asci and these are known as paraphyses (singular – paraphysis). Ascospores vary greatly in size, from minute to more than 1000µm in length, in shape from thread-like to globose, and from hyaline to black and from one to many-celled. These characteristics are used as criteria in the classification.

Ascocarps: Ascomycetes produce their asci in the fruiting bodies known as ascocarps. In general, the classification of the class is based according to the manner in which the asci are borne and are generally divided into four major categories.

1. Those which produce their asci inside and completely closed ascocarp is known as 'Cleistothecium'.

2. Those which produce their asci in a much less closed structure but provided with a small opening or hole through which the ascospores are liberated at maturity. This structure is called a 'Perithecium'.

3. Those fungi which produce asci in an open ascocarp termed 'Apothecium'.

In addition to these three types of ascocarps, there are various modifications resulting in the production of a number of intermediate forms.

Ex: Ascocarp and ascogenous hyphae absent the members bear naked asci - Taphrinales

Taphrina deformans - Peach leaf curl

T. maculans - Leaf blotch of turmeric

Asci can be clearly seen in section of diseased leaves from the exposed layer. Initially there are eight ascospores. These ascospores produce secondary spores called conidia by budding. A small out-growth known as bud develops at one end of the cell. As the bud enlarges, the nucleus divides by the process of direct division and the daughter nuclei pass into the bud. The bud gradually grows bigger and finally separates from the mother cell.

Sexual Reproduction

Nuclear fusion occurs between two somatic cells or two ascospores which assume the function of copulating gametangia and a zygote cell results finally producing ascospores.

Life Cycle of *Erysiphe cichoracearum* Causing Powdery Mildew in Cucurbits

Division: Eumycota

Sub-Division: Ascomycotina

Class: Plectomycetes

Order: Erysiphales

Family: Erysiphaceae

Genus: *Erysiphe*

Species: *E. cichoracearum*

The fungus produces abundant superficial mycelium which forms a white coating over the leaf. The white growth consists of mycelium, conidiophores and conidia. The fungus remains superficially on the leaf surface and sends only haustoria into the epidermal cells. The fungal growth is generally seen on the upper

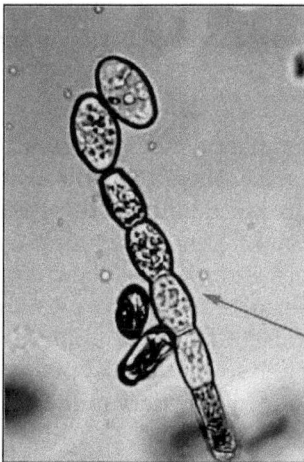

Figure 23: Conidiophore with Conidial Chain of *Erysiphe* spp.

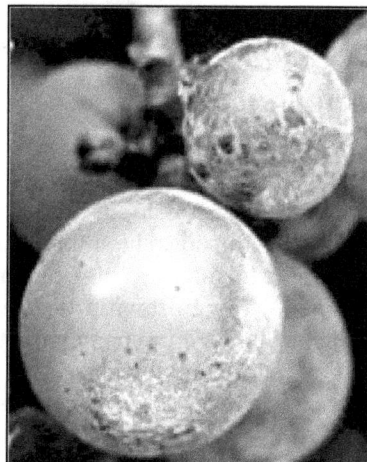

Figure 24: Powdery Mildew on Grapes.

surface of the leaves and very often the entire leaf is involved in the attack. As a result of the infection, the leaves dry up and soon fall off. In severe cases, heavy defoliation occurs and this results in the stunted growth of the plant.

Asexual Reproduction

A few days after infection a large number of hyaline, erect conidiophores begin to develop on the superficial mycelium. Conidia cut off one below the other at the tips of the conidiophores. The entire conidiophore with conidia will be seen in the form of a basipetal chain with the oldest conidium at the top. These conidia are uninucleate, hyaline, one-celled and capable of remaining in a viable state only for a short time. They are easily carried by wind and under favorable conditions germinate producing germ tube which develops into a mycelium (The imperfect or asexual stage is *Oidium* spp.).

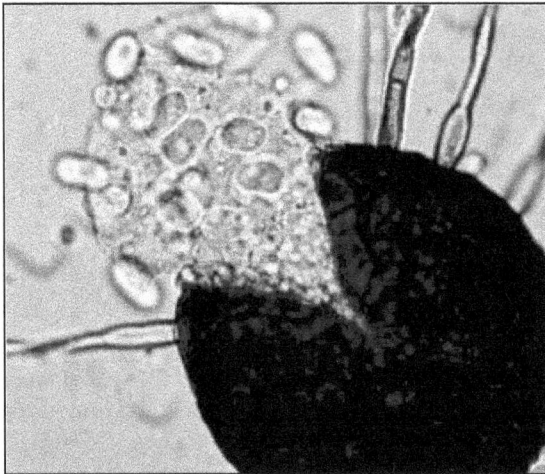

Figure 25: Cleistothecium with Asci and Ascospores of *Erysiphe* spp.

Sexual Reproduction

After a period of vegetative activity the conidial production slows down and eventually ceases. Young cleisto-thecia appear on the whitish superficial mycelium. The uninucleate gametangia (antheridium and ascogonium) arise from closely situated hyphal threads. The antheridium is somewhat slender than the asco-gonium and they apply themselves close together. The formation of cleistothecium and ascus development is long drawn processes. The cleistothecia have very characteristic appendages. This genus has characteristic coiled tips to the appendages. The ascospores get liberated from asci on maturity and infect the host plant to initiate new infection. This type of life cycle is common in all powdery mildews.

Comparison of Downy Mildews and Powdery Mildews

Sl.No.	Downy Mildews	Powdery Mildews
1.	Mostly seen on the lower surface of the leaves, with a corresponding yellow patch on the other side of the leaf	Generally seen on the upper surface of the leaf
2.	The growth is soft and whiter	The growth is powdery and dull white
3.	The downy growth consists of sporangiophore and sporangia	The powdery growth consists of mycelium, conidio-phores and conidia
4.	Mycelium coenocytic	Mycelium septate.
5.	Fungi belong to Mastigomycotina	Fungi belong to Ascomycotina
6.	Sexual spores - Oospores	Ascospores in cleistothecia
7.	Motile spores - Present (zoospores)	Motile spores – Absent
8.	Antheridium and Oogonium	Antheridium and Ascogonium
9.	Common during high humid weather	Common during dry season
10.	Endophytic	Ectophytic or Endophytic

Division: Eumycota

Sub-Division-4: BASIDIOMYCOTINA

This sub-division comprises of a large number of higher fungi. The true Basidiomycotina consists of forms like mushroom, toadstool, puffballs and stink horns. The so-called shell or Bracket fungi and Bird's nest fungi also belong to this group. The smuts, the rusts and the jelly fungi also belong to Basidiomycotina. This sub-division differs from others in that they produce the spores called basidiospores externally on the specialised spore-bearing structure called basidium. A typical basidium produces four one-celled haploid uninucleate spores. The hyphae of the mycelium are highly septate and penetrate into the substratum to absorb nourishment. It is usually white, light yellow or orange in colour. In some forms they produce thick strands called rhizomorphs. The mycelium passes through three distinct stages of development before the fungus completes its life cycle; primary mycelium, secondary mycelium and tertiary mycelium. The primary mycelium develops from germination of basidiospore. The secondary mycelium originates from the primary mycelium. Its cells are typically binucleate. Clamp connections are present. The tertiary mycelium is represented by specialised tissues which compose the sporophores. The cells of this mycelium are binucleate. Thus the basidium, the presence of dikaryotic mycelium and the formation of clamp connections are the typical characteristics of this sub-division. The basidia are typically formed in definite layers called hymeneal layer. In the hymeneal layer, some sterile structure much larger than basidia, called cystidia are seen mixed with basidia.

The basidium originates from a terminal cell of a binucleate mycelium and is separated by a septum. The two nuclei in the young basidium fuse and the zygote nucleus undergoes reduction division giving rise to four haploid nuclei. In the meantime four sterigmata are pushed out at the top of the basidium and their tips enlarge forming basidiospore initials. The 4 nuclei now squeeze through the sterigmatal passage into the young basidiospores which eventually develop as uninucleate haploid basidiospores.

Life Cycle of *Gymnosporangium juniperi-virginianae* Causing Rust of Apple

Division: Eumycota

Sub-Division: Basidiomycotina

Class: Basidiomycetes

Order: Uredinales

Family: Pucciniaceae

Genus: *Gymnosporangium*

Species: *G. juniperi-virginianae*

The fungus cycles between primary host, eastern red cedar and its alternate host either apple or crab apple. The pathogen over-winters as teliospores in horn-like telia on eastern red cedar. During rainy period, the telia become swollen and turn into gelatinous mass and again drying back to dark brown threads. During rain induced swelling, some of the teliospores are exuded which germinate to produce basidium. However, all the teliospores present in a horn do not germinate at the same time. One horn may undergo number of periods of gelatinization and teliospores germinate during the spring resulting in continuous supply of basidiospores during the entire period of apple flowering and generating new leaves. Basidiospores are forcibly discharged into the air immediately after formation and can be carried by air currents.

The basidiospores, on reaching young apple leaves, germinate in a water film and infect the host tissues. Subsequently, flask shaped spermagonia of rust develop on apple leaves and fruits in the spring. After two weeks, orange-brown pycnia containing pycniospores appear on the upper side of the leaves or fruits. Young leaves 4-8 days old are highly susceptible and fruits are vulnerable from tight cluster stage until just after petal fall. Two months after appearance of pycnia, aecia appear on the lower surface of leaves or fruits. The aecia produce aeciospores, which are released during dry weather in late summer and infect young needles or auxiliary buds of eastern red cedar.

The pathogen survives the winter as dikaryotic mycelium in the tissues of the junipers. In the next year after infection, galls are formed which produce teliospores during the spring only. Fresh infections of eastern red cedar are required each year for infection of apple trees. The telial galls are produced on cedar which cause dieback of small branches. Wet weather conditions are necessary for gelatination of telial horns and germination of teliospores. This process require about 4-6 hours after wetting. Wind currents are also required for dissemination of basidiospores. The degree of infection further depends upon topography and direction of orchard and velocity of wind.

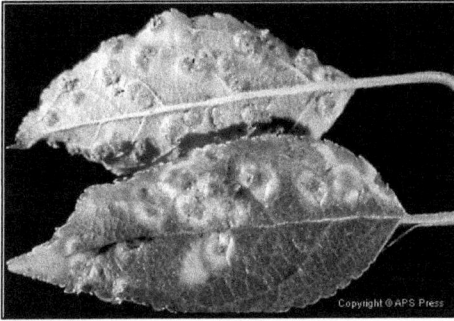

| Apple leaves with spermagonia and aecia | Cross section of leaf |

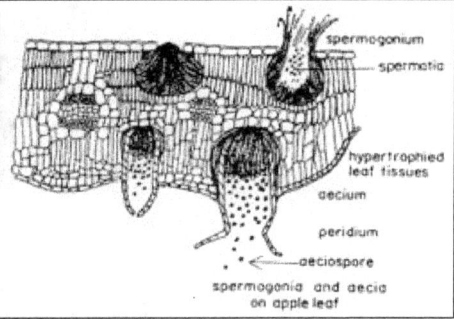

Figure 26: Cedar-Apple Rust.

Life Cycle of *Ganoderma lucidum* Causing Basal Stem Rot (Root Rot and Wilt) of Palms

Division: Eumycota

Sub-Division: Basidiomycotina

Class: Hymenomycetes

Order: Aphyllophorales

Genus: *Ganodcrma*

Species: *G. lucidum*

This fungus causes wilt or root-rot diseases on palms mainly Coconut, oil palm and Arecanut. It also infects several other horticultural crops and forest trees. In the affected plants, the leaves change in colour from dark green to dull green. Later, they droop down as if they are suffering from lack of water. The crown shrinks and central core of the stem becomes soft and rotten resulting in the collapse of the plant. Sometimes a colored fluid also oozes out through natural cracks at the base of the stem. The organism lives in top soil. The vegetative mycelium is profusely branched and provided with clamp connections. The mycelium spreads in the soil and the trees are infected through roots. The fructifications or the fruiting bodies of the fungus appear at the base of the affected plant at a later stage. The fruiting body is a bracket-shaped structure. Their lateral and upper surfaces are coated with hard shining substances. This structure is woody in texture and its size varies from 1" to 20" in diameter and about 4-5" thickness.

The upper surface of the bracket is the pileus and it is slimy dark brown to almost black in colour with concentric furrows. The margins will be generally white in colour. When the bracket is closely examined a large number of minute pores are seen on the under surface of the brackets. These pores represent the openings of the numerous hymenial tubes which are vertically oriented and serve as the exit points for the basidiospores. The inner surfaces of hymenial tubes are lined with basidia which bear basidiospores and these are borne on sterigmata. The basidiospores are brown in colour and peculiar in shape having two knob-like projections at the base.

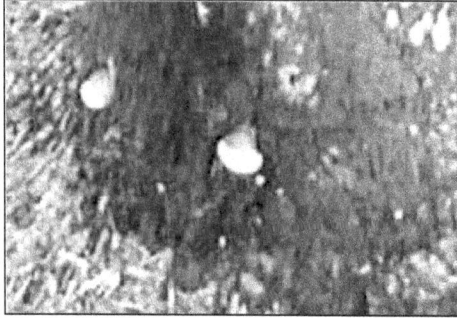

Brackets on base of the stem

Figure 27: Basal Stem Rot of Coconut.

Division: Eumycota

Sub-Division-5: DEUTEROMYCOTINA

The Fungi Imperfecti or imperfect fungi, also known as Deuteromycota are fungi which do not fit into the commonly established taxonomic classifications of fungi that are based on biological species, concepts or morphological characteristics of sexual structures because their sexual form of reproduction has never been observed; hence the name "imperfect fungi". Only their asexual form of reproduction is known, meaning that this group of fungus produces their spores asexually.

The *Deuteromycota* (Greek for "second fungi") were once considered a formal phylum of the Fungi. The term is now used only informally, to denote species of fungi that are asexually reproducing members of the fungal phyla Ascomycota and Basidiomycota.

1. The Sub-Division Deuteromycotina includes fungi having septate mycelium, which reproduce only by asexual methods.

2. Mycelium is well-developed, septate with branched hyphae. These are multinucleate.

3. All the members (except 1 group) reproduce asexually by means of special spores known as conidia.

4. A conidium is a non-motile, asexual spore formed at the tip or side of a sporongenous cell called conidiophore.

5. These fungi lack sexual or perfect stage, hence, commonly called as "Imperfect fungi" or more technically "Fungi Imperfecti".

6. The conidia produced by these fungi resemble the conidia of ascomycotina.

7. The mycelium of these fungi sporulates rather rapidly in culture as well as in nature.

8. The factors inducing sporulation have been studied (Temperature, nutrition, light and pH).

9. Sporulation in the Deuteromycetes is strictly an asexual process.

10. Since present classification is based on characters of sexual stage, these fungi are not fit for the classification.

11. Accordingly all these fungi are grouped into a Sub-Division Deuteromycotina, which is sub-divided into Form, orders, families, genera and species.

Criteria for Classification of Deuteromycotina

1. Presence or absence of asexual spores.
2. Type of asexual fruiting body.
3. Manner of production of asexual spores.
4. Size, shape, color and septation of asexual spores.

According to Ainsworth (1973), Deuteromycotina is divided into 3 form classes 1) Coelomycetes 2) Hyphomycetes and 3) Blastomycetes.

Life Cycle of *Colletotrichum capsici* Causing Die-back and Fruit Rot in Chillies

> Division: Eumycota
>
> Sub-Division: Deuteromycotina
>
> Class: Coelomycetes
>
> Order: Melanconiales
>
> Family: Melanconiaceae
>
> Genus: *Colletotrichum*
>
> Species: *C. capsici*

This fungus causes a serious disease on chillies called 'die-back and fruit-rot'. The disease generally appears during months between October and December. When the crop approaches maturity, indivi-dual flowers are found drooping and gradually drying up. Many of them fall off.

Under favorable conditions the infection spreads to the stem through flower stalk and causes 'die-back' of the branches and stem. In this manner the entire upper portion of the plant may get killed.

The disease is very severe on the fruits. Ripening fruits are more liable to attack than the green ones. Brown water-soaked patches appear on the skin of the fruits. As the disease progresses the patches increase in size and the entire fruit is involved in the attack. As a result the whole fruit shrivels and dries up. Such fruits become white in color and lose their pungency. On the surfaces of the affected fruits minute black structures called acervuli appear in large numbers. Each acervulus consists of a stroma, setae (stiff black sterile hairy structures), non-septate, short hyaline conidiophores and sickle or cresent-shaped conidia. Acervuli are sometimes formed on the seed as black dots.

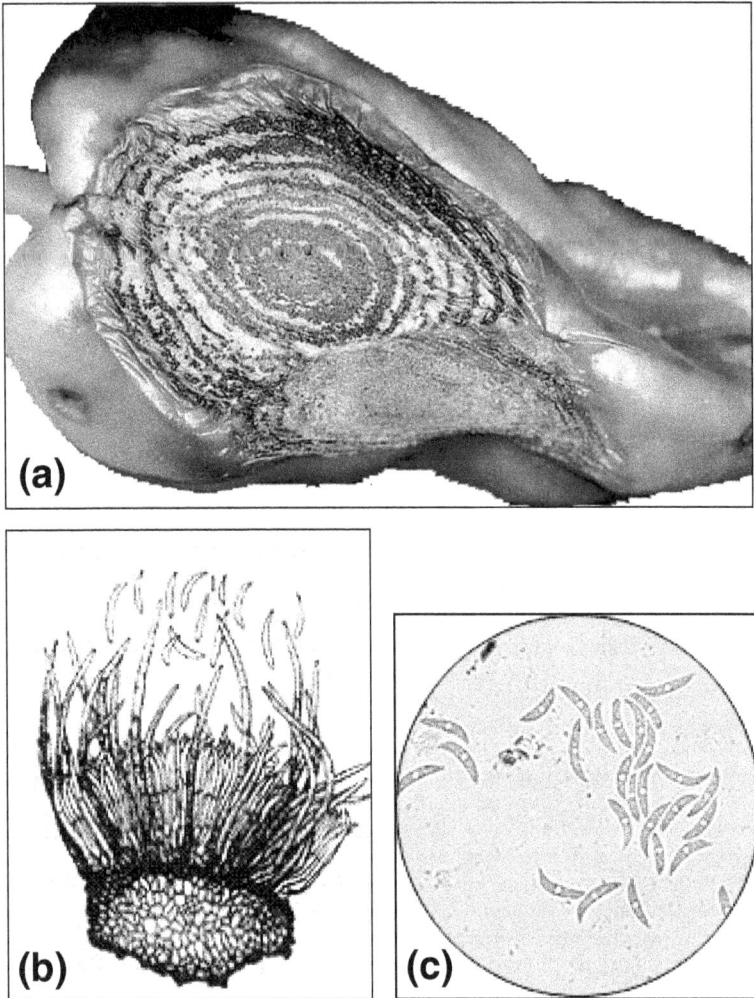

Figure 28: *Colletotrichum capsici*
(a) Infection on Chilli Fruits, (b) Acervulus, (c) Conidia.

Mycelium is highly septate and profusely branched. From the internal hyphae stromata are formed on the epidermis or just below the epidermis. They increase in size and rupture the cuticle and then continue to grow so as to form a cushion-shaped structure on the surface. The surface cells of the stroma grow out into two kinds of stalks. Some stalks grow into long dark, rigid sterile hairs called setae while between them others grow into hyaline short, closely crowded stalks called conidiophores. The conidiophores bear conidia at their tips. The conidia are borne singly on non-septate unbranched conidiophores. The spore mass is pink in color but the conidia are hyaline individually. The conidia are non-septate, curved (sickle-shaped), and narrowed at the ends. On germination a germ tube is given out from one or both the ends. Appressoria are formed at the ends of these germ tubes and infection takes place usually by hyphal thread from the appressorium. The sexual state is not known.

Life Cycle of *Septoria lycopersici* Causing *Septoria* Leaf Spot on Tomato

Division: Eumycota

Sub-Division: Deuteromycotina

Class: Coelomycetes

Order: Sphaeropsidales

Family: Sphaeropsidaceae

Genus: *Septoria*

Species: *S. lycopersici*

The members of this genus cause some important crop diseases like leaf spot on tomato caused by *Septoria lycopersici* and leaf spot on celery caused by *S. apii.*

The disease on tomato is characterized by the formation of spots on the leaves and sometimes on the leaf stalks also. Under favorable conditions, heavy spotting of the leaves occur resulting in stunted growth of the plant. On the spots the fructifications of the fungus appear in the form of black dots. They may appear on both the sides of affected leaf. The mycelium consists of brown-colored intercellular hyphae. The fructification is a flask shaped structure with an outer dark colored wall called peridium. The structure opens to outside by means of a small hole, called 'ostiole', at its tip. The entire structure is called pycnidium. Lining the inner walls of the pycnidia, a layer of cells giving rise to short straight simple conidiophores bearing needle-shaped straight or slightly curved septate conidia arise. The spores are discharged through the ostiole in a mucilaginous mass. Under favorable conditions, the spores germinate producing a germ tube and new infection occurs through the stomatal opening. The perfect stages of the fungus very often belong to the genera *Mycosphaerella, Leptosphaeria* of the order *Sphaeriales* under the sub-division *Ascomycotina*.

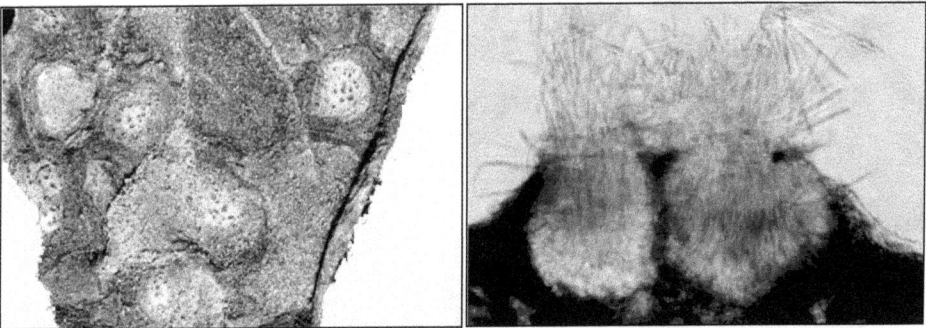

Figure 29: *Septoria lycopersici* Infection on Leaf and Pycnidia with Conidia.

Life Cycle of *Alternaria solani* Causing Early Blight of Potato and Tomato

Division: Eumycota

Sub-Division: Deuteromycotina

Class: Dothideomycetes

Family: Pleosporaccae

Genus: *Alternaria*

Species: *A. solani*

There are 299 species in the genus. They are ubiquitous in the environment and are a natural part of fungal flora almost everywhere. They are normal agents of decay and decomposition. At least 20 per cent of agricultural spoilage is caused by *Alternaria* species. Many human health disorders can be caused by these fungi, which grow on skin and mucous membranes, including on the eyeballs and within the respiratory tract. The terms *alternariosis* and *alternaria toxicosis* are used for disorders in humans and animals caused by a fungus in this genus.

Several members of the genus *Alternaria* are pathogens on several economic crops causing losses in quality and quantity of the produce. Some of them are *A. solani* – causes early blight in potatoes and tomatoes; *A. alternata* – besides causing blight on several plant species including potato, it also causes upper respiratory infections in AIDS patients, asthma in people with sensitivity, and has been implicated in chronic rhinosinusitis; *A. arborescens* – causes canker of tomato; *A. brassicae* – infects many roses and many vegetables; *A. brassicicola* and *A. japonica* – infect crucifers and *A. dauci* – infects carrots.

Alternaria solani survives the winter either in the soil or plant debris or as conidia from other hosts. When the potato foliage comes in contact with the contaminated soil or plant debris it forms a lesion. This lesion then produces spores which are responsible for secondary infection. Spore formation is optimal with foliage that

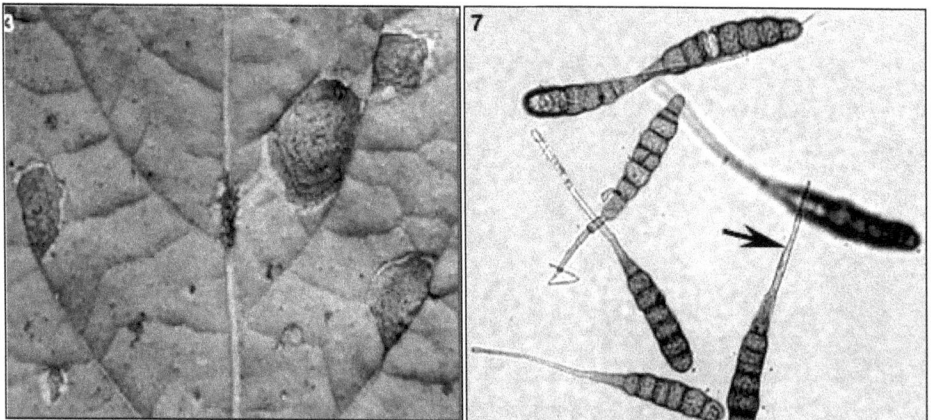

Figure 30: *Alternaria solani* Infection on Potato and Conidia of *A. solani*.

alternates between wet and dry conditions. Such is the case with overhead irrigation systems or frequent dew or fog. Spores that are formed can be dislodged by wind and rain and are carried to foliage and soil within that field as well as to surrounding fields. Infection spreads to tubers through wounds during or after harvest. This occurs when a wounded tuber comes in contact with contaminated soil or plant material. Moisture on tuber surfaces and warm environments help favor infection. At the end of the season, the fungus reaches the soil to survive during off-season either in the soil as saprophyte or on plant debris as dormant mycelium till next crop season.

Division: Eumycota

Sub-Division: Deuteromycotina

Class: Coelomycetes

Order: Aganomycetales

All members of the Sub-Division Deuteromycotina whose conidial stages are not known are classified under this order. It is not divided into families as no definite basis for the classification could be recognised. The group receives its name from the fact that no spores or fruiting bodies are formed by the members. Some of them form sclerotia, which are compact structures of definite form usually light coloured internally but bearing a dark tough rind outside. *Sclerotium rolfsii* and *S. oryzae* are important in the genus *Sclerotium*. Another genus *Rhizoctonia* is equally important, causing several plant diseases. *R. solani* is a very important plant pathogen with characteristic coarse septate hyphae and having lateral branches constricted at the point of origin.

Life Cycle of *Sclerotium rolfsii* Causing Blights, Cankers, Rots and Wilts of a wide Variety of both Food Crops and Ornamental Plants

The diseases caused by Sclerotium rolfsii are serious problems for both agriculture and the nursery industry, and is very hard to eradicate once established in a garden. The disease affects a wide variety of field crops like cotton, tobacco, soybean, peanuts, maize; fruit and plantation crops like mango, banana, coffee, pineapple, vegetables like onion, garlic, carrot, celery, beet, brassicas, pepper, lettuce, cucurbits, tomato, potato, brinjal, beans, peas, colocasia, cucumber, yam, and ginger; ornamental plants like chrysanthemum, carnations, *Hibiscus*, *Ipomoea*, cherrys, tuberose, tulip, and weed plants like *Cynadon*. Southern blight is the name given to the disease on cucurbits (pumpkins and squash) caused by *S. rolfsii*.

As the fungus is known to produce sclerotia, it is placed under imperfect fungi. However, in recent years the sexual stages of the fungus were discovered and have been placed under Basidiomycotina. As such, it has several synonyms and classified under different families. The synonyms are *Sclerotium delphini* (A); *Corticium rolfsii* (T); *Athelia rolfsii* (T) and *Pellicularia rolfsii* (T).

Classification	Athelia rolfsii	Corticium rolfsii	Sclerotium rolfsii
Division	Eumycota	Eumycota	Eumycota
Sub-division	Basidiomycotina	Basidiomycotina	Basidiomycotina
Class	Hymenomycetes	Hymenomycetes	Hymenomycetes
Order	Polyporales	Polyporales	Agaricales
Family	Atheliaceae	Corticiaceae	Typhulaceae
Genus	Athelia	Corticium	Sclerotium
Species	A. rolfsii	C. rolfsii	S. rolfsii

Initial southern blight infections arise from sclerotia which overwinter in the fields. Sclerotia of the fungus are similar to seeds of a plant in that they remain dormant until conditions become favorable for germination. Conditions that favor germination and infection are high moisture, warm to hot temperatures, and the presence of dead plant litter on the soil surface. Moisture requirements can be met from irrigation or rainfall. Decaying plant debris or weed residues stimulate germination of sclerotia and serve as a food base for the fungus. The fungus then grows outward from the food sources and infects any part of the crop in contact with the soil surface. Plant tissues are killed by an acid produced by the fungus. Disease development below the soil surface can be extensive in sandy, well-aerated soils resulting in severe rot. When plants are killed and the food supply of the fungus becomes limiting, numerous sclerotia develop that easily dislodge and fall to the soil surface. Sclerotia survive well at the soil surface but survive poorly when buried deep because the fungus has a high demand for oxygen. Sclerotia at or near the soil surface can survive three to four years, while survival is a year or less when sclerotia are buried deeply.

The southern blight fungus does not produce spores which move in the air, so the disease is confined to localized areas in a field where sclerotia occur. Centers of disease are numerous where high numbers of sclerotia are distributed near the soil surface and conditions are favorable for southern blight. The occurrence and severity of southern blight epidemics are difficult to predict because of interactions between numbers of sclerotia near the soil surface, moisture and temperature levels, amount of plant residue, and canopy density.

Management

1. Practice crop rotation with non-susceptible crops such as sorghum, pearl millet etc.
2. Moldboard plow to bury sclerotia and crop residue deep into the soil.
3. Plant on a raised bed to improve drainage and reduce levels of moisture in the canopy.
4. Apply fungicides like pentachloro nitrobenzene (PCNB) to reduce losses when southern blight is a main factor limiting production.
5. Time irrigations to apply adequate but not excessive amounts of water and avoid frequently applying small amounts of water.

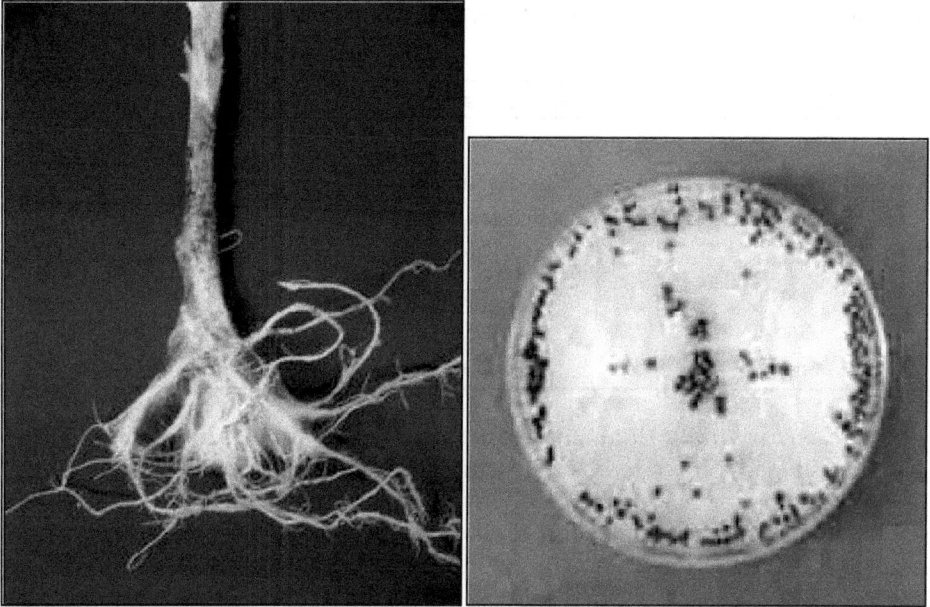

Figure 31: *Sclerotium rolfsii* **Infected Potato Stem and Sclerotia in Culture.**

6. Maintain foliar disease control to reduce accumulation of leaf litter in the soil near the base of the plants.

Life Cycle of *Rhizoctonia solani* Causing Damping Off in many Crops and Wire Stem in Cabbage, Cauliflower and related Plants

Rhizoctonia solani is a plant pathogenic fungus with a wide host range and worldwide distribution. It is one cause of the condition known as damping off, which is a cause of death of seedlings in agriculture. It is also responsible for wire stem, a disease of cabbage, cauliflower and related plants that is similar to damping off but attacks older seedlings and produces a constricted, wiry stem. It does not produce spores and is hence identified only from mycelial characteristics. Its hyphal cells are multinucleate. It produces white to deep brown mycelium when grown on artificial medium. The hyphae are 4-15 µm wide and tend to branch at right angles. A septum near each hyphal branch and a slight constriction at the branch are diagnostic. *R. solani* is sub-divided into anastomosis groups (AG) based on hyphal fusion between compatible strains.

R. solani can infect several field crops like rice, maize, soybean, sorghum, tobacco, cotton, flax and wheat; vegetables like bean, cabbage, lettuce, carrot, crucifers, ginger, onion, pea, and sugar beet; and ornamentals like gladiolus, chrysanthemum and tulips.

The teleomorph of *R. solani* is *Thanatephorus cucumeris*. It forms club-shaped basidia with four apical sterigmata on which oval, hyaline basidiospores are borne.

It is having about 50 synonyms. The systematic position for these two forms is tabulated here.

Classification	Rhizoctonia solani	Thanatephorus cucumeris
Division	Eumycota	Eumycota
Sub-division	Basidiomycotina	Basidiomycotina
Class	Hymenomycetes	Hymenomycetes
Order	Polyporales	Ceratobasidiales
Family	Corticiaceae	Ceratobasidiaceae
Genus	*Rhizoctonia*	*Thanatephorus*
Species	*R. solani*	*T. cucumeris*

R. solani can survive for many years by producing small (1 to 3 mm diameter), irregular-shaped, brown to black structures (called sclerotia) in soil and on plant tissue. Certain rice pathogens of *R. solani*, have evolved the ability to produce sclerotia with a thick outer layer that allows them to float and survive in water. *R. solani* also survives as mycelium by colonizing soil organic matter as a saprophyte, particularly as a result of plant pathogenic activity. Sclerotia and/or mycelium present in soil and/or on plant tissue germinate to produce vegetative threads (hyphae) of the fungus that can attack a wide range of food and fiber crops.

The fungus is attracted to the plant by chemical stimulants released by actively growing plant cells and/or decomposing plant residues. As the attraction process proceeds, the fungal hypha will come in contact with the plant and become attached to its external surface. After attachment, the fungus continues to grow on the external surface of the plant and will cause disease by producing a specialized infection structure (either an appressorium or infection cushion) that penetrates the plant cell and releases nutrients for continued fungal growth and development. The infection process is promoted by the production of many different extracellular enzymes that degrade various components of plant cell walls (*e.g.* cellulose, cutin and pectin). As the fungus kills the plant cells, the hyphae continue to grow and colonize dead tissue, often forming sclerotia. New inoculum is produced on or in host tissue, and a new cycle is repeated when new substrates become available.

Management

1. Practice crop rotation with non-susceptible crops.
2. Plough to bury sclerotia and crop residue deep into the soil.
3. Plant on a raised bed to improve drainage and reduce levels of moisture in the canopy.
4. Apply fungicides like pentachloro nitrobenzene (PCNB) or chlorothalonil or mancozeb or thiophanate methyl to reduce losses when southern blight is a main factor limiting production.
5. Time irrigations to apply adequate but not excessive amounts of water and avoid frequently applying small amounts of water.

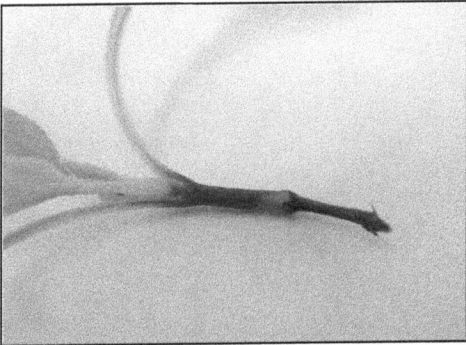

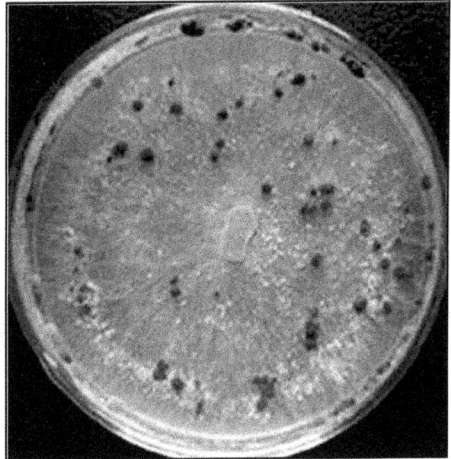

Figure 32: *Rhizoctonia solani* Infection on Crucifers causing Wirestem and Damping Off; and Sclerotia in Culture.

6. Maintain foliar disease control to reduce accumulation of leaf litter in the soil near the base of the plants.

6

General Account of Phytopathogenic Bacteria

Many economically-important diseases of plants are caused by members of the Bacteria. It is estimated that one-eighth of the crops worldwide are lost due to diseases caused by bacteria, fungi or insects. Almost all kinds of plants can be affected by bacterial diseases, and many of these diseases can be extremely destructive.

Bacteriology

It is a science which deals with the study of bacteria.

Phytopathogenic Bacteria

The bacteria that cause disease in plants.

Bacteria can be defined as *"Extremely minute, rigid, essentially unicellular organisms, free of true chlorophyll and generally devoid of any photosynthetic pigment, most commonly multiplying asexually by simple transverse binary fission with the resulting cells nearly equal in size"*.

In order to be able to colonise the plant they have specific pathogenicity factors. Five main types of bacterial pathogenicity factors are known:

1. *Cell wall degrading enzymes* - Used to break down the plant cell wall in order to release the nutrients inside by pathogens such as *Erwinia* to cause soft-rot.

2. *Toxins* - These can be non-host specific, and damage all plants, or host-specific and only cause damage on a host plant.

3. *Effector proteins* - These can be secreted into the extracellular environment or directly into the host cell, often via the Type three secretion system, *i.e.*, an organelle, (a protein structure) used to secrete proteins that help the bacteria infect multicellular, eukaryotic organisms. Some effectors are known to suppress host defense processes.

4. *Phytohormones* - For example, *Agrobacterium* changes the level of Auxin to cause tumours.

5. *Exopolysaccharides* - These are produced by bacteria and block xylem vessels, often leading to wilting and death of the plant.

Bacteria controls the production of pathogenicity factors via quorum sensing, *i.e.*, coordinate their gene expression according to the local density of their population.

Thomas J. Burrill (1839-1916) of USA was the first person to relate bacterium as a cause of plant disease. He worked on fire blight of apples and pears and proved *Erwinia amylovora* as the cause of disease in 1878.

General Characters of Phytopathogenic Bacteria

1. Prokaryotic, unicellular, heterotrophic micro-organism.

2. Genome: A large circular chromosome composed of DNA.

3. Presence of rigid cell wall with capsule (or) slime layer.

4. Majority are Gram negative except Clavibacter (Corynebacterium) and Streptomyces which are Gram positive.

5. Majority are rods except Streptomyces (filamentous).

6. None of the phytopathogenic bacteria forms endospores.

7. Majority are flagellate, hence, motile.

8. All are capable of living as saprophytes, hence can be cultured in laboratory.

9. All are susceptible to phages.

10. Majority are aerobic except *Erwinia* which is facultative anaerobic (*Cornybacter*).

11. Reproduction is by simple transverse Binary fission.

12. Requires incubation for 48 hours at 25°C for initial growth.

Classification of 'Phytopathogenic Bacteria'

Kingdom Procaryotae

Bacteria – Have cell membrane and cell wall

I) Division: Gracilicutes – Gram-negative bacteria

a) Class: Proteobacteria – Mostly single-celled bacteria

i) Family: Enterobacteriaceae

Genus: *Erwinia*, causing fire blight of Pear and apple

ii) Family: Pseudomonadaceae

Genus: *Pseudomonas,* causing numerous Leaf spots, blights, vascular wilts, soft rots, cankers, and galls

Ralstonia causing wilts of solanaceous crops

Rhizobacter causing the bacterial gall of carrot

Rhizomonas causing the corky root rot of lettuce

Xanthomonas causing numerous leaf spots, fruit spots, and blights of annual and perennial plants, vascular wilts, and citrus canker

Xylophilus causing the bacterial necrosis and canker of grapevines

iii) Family: Burkholderiaceae

Genus: *Burkholderia:* Gram –ve group of bacteria which includes animal, human and plant pathogens as well as some environmentally-important species. The genus was named after Walter H. Burkholder, plant pathologist who discovered that sour skin of onions is caused by *Pseudomonas cepacia* (now *Burkholderria cepacia*).

iv) Family: Ralstoniaceae

Genus: *Ralstonia:* Gram-negative, plant pathogenic, soil bacterium

v) Family: Rhizobiaceae

Genus: *Agrobacterium,* the cause of Crown gall disease

Rhizobium, the cause of root nodules in legumes

vi) Family: still unnamed

Genus: *Xylella,* xylem–inhabiting, causing leaf scorch and dieback diseases on trees and vines

Liberobacter, phloem inhabiting, causing citrus greening disease

II) Division: Firmicutes – Gram-positive bacteria

a) Class: Firmibacteria-Mostly single-celled bacteria.

Genus: *Bacillus,* causing rot of tubers, seeds, and seedlings

Clostridium, causing rot of stored tubers and leaves and wet wood of elm and poplars

b) Class: Thallobacteria – Branching bacteria

Genus: *Clavibacter,* causing bacterial wilts in alfalfa, potato, and tomato

Streptomyces, causing the common potato scab

III) Division: Tenericutes

a) Class: Mollicutes - Have only cell membrane and lack cell wall

i) Family: Spiroplasmataceae

Genus: *Spiroplasma,* causing citrus stubborn disease

ii) Family(ies): still unknown

Genus: *Phytoplasma*, causing numerous yellows, proliferation, and decline in trees and some annuals.

Key to different Phytopathogenic Bacteria

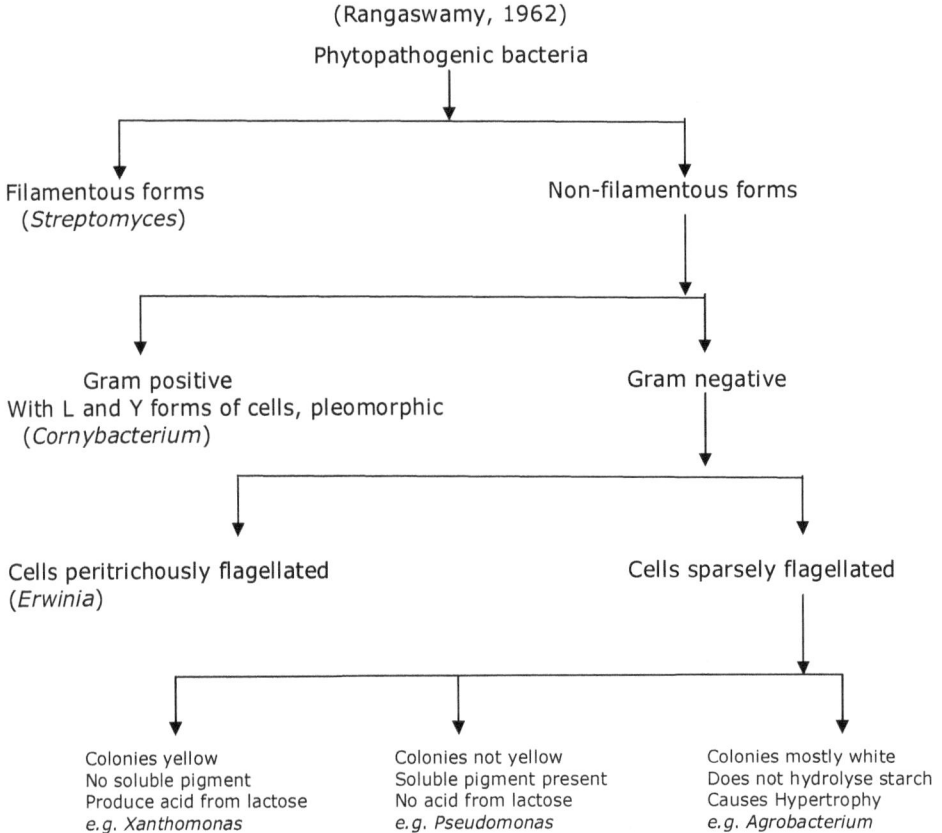

(Rangaswamy, 1962)

Phytopathogenic bacteria

Filamentous forms
(*Streptomyces*)

Non-filamentous forms

Gram positive
With L and Y forms of cells, pleomorphic
(*Cornybacterium*)

Gram negative

Cells peritrichously flagellated
(*Erwinia*)

Cells sparsely flagellated

Colonies yellow
No soluble pigment
Produce acid from lactose
e.g. Xanthomonas

Colonies not yellow
Soluble pigment present
No acid from lactose
e.g. Pseudomonas

Colonies mostly white
Does not hydrolyse starch
Causes Hypertrophy
e.g. Agrobacterium

Important Characters of 'Phytopathogenic Genera' of Bacteria

Agrobacterium

☆ Cells are rod-shaped.

☆ Motile by 1-4 peritrichous flagella.

☆ If only 1 flagellum is present it is lateral than polar.

☆ Colonies are non-pigmented and smooth.

☆ Bacteria are soil and rhizosphere inhabitants.

☆ Forms galls in plants.

Clavibacter (Corynebacterium)

☆ Cells are rod-shaped, straight or slightly curved.

☆ Also exhibit club-shaped forms.

☆ Also exhibit angular attachment and palisade appearance.

☆ Chemo-organotrophs, facultative anaerobic.

☆ Gram +ve.

☆ These may have 1-3 polar or sub-polar flagella.

Erwinia

☆ Cell single and straight rods.

☆ Motile by peritrichous flagella.

☆ Gram -ve, facultative anaerobes.

☆ Associated with plants either as pathogens or as saprophytes.

Pseudomonas

☆ Cells single, straight or curved rods but not helical.

☆ Motile by polar flagella.

☆ Mono or Lophotrichous.

☆ Gram -ve, chemo-organotrophs and strictly aerobic.

☆ Cultures may or may not produce water-soluble bluish, greenish or brown fluorescent pigments.

Burkholderia

☆ Gram-negative.

☆ Motile by polar flagella.

☆ Obligately aerobic.

☆ Rod-shaped.

☆ Until very recently classified as *Pseudomonas*, these resemble the latter in most respects with the important difference that its cells do not produce fluorescent pigments.

Ralstonia

☆ Aerobic.

☆ Non-spore forming.

☆ Gram-negative.

☆ Rodshaped.

☆ Motile with a polar flagellar tuft.

☆ Until very recently classified as *Pseudomonas*, these resemble the latter in most respects with the important difference that its cells do not produce fluorescent pigments.

Xanthomonas

☆ Cells single, straight rods.

☆ Motile by means of polar flagella.

☆ Sheaths and resting spores are not produced.

☆ Gram –ve.

☆ Grows on cultural medium which is usually yellow in colour.

☆ Chemo-organotrophs and strictly aerobic.

☆ Cultures develop yellow, non-water soluble pigments.

Streptomyces

☆ Cells are spherical to avoid.

☆ Occur in pairs, occasionally in chains.

☆ Produce motile strains.

☆ Gram +ve.

☆ Facultative anaerobic.

☆ Chemo-organotrophs.

☆ Conidia are produced in chains (No such conidia in nocardia).

Important Diseases Caused by Phytopathogenic Bacteria, their Symptoms and Management

Citrus Canker

Causal Organism: *Xanthomonas axonopodis* p.v. citri

Symptoms

On leaves: Small yellowish spots on leaves – spots swell and raised above the surface as brown corky outgrowth or spongy eruption – spots are surrounded by yellow halo.

On twigs: Irregular raised cankers on the surface.

On fruits: Round to irregular raised cankerous growth on the surface. The cankerous spots are few to many. Cankers usually coalesce.

Management

☆ Spraying with Bordeaux mixture (2:2:250), streptomycin or Agrimycin-100 @ 150 mg/ml reduces the disease.

☆ Pruning and destruction of diseased plants minimized the disease.

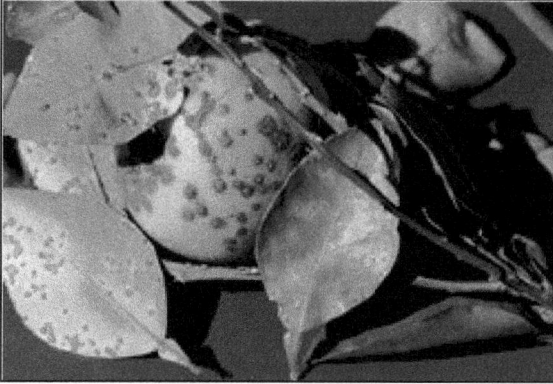

Figure 33: Citrus Canker on Leaves and Fruits.

Fire Blight of Apple

Causal Organism: *Erwinia amylovora.*

Symptoms

Blossoms first appear water-soaked, then shrivel, wilt and turn brownish to black. After the blossoms, the succulent twigs or shoots and water-sprouts or suckers are the next most susceptible parts of the plant. Fruit blight symptoms are common in immature fruits. Infection spreads through lenticels, wounds or from infected spurs into the fruit. Infected apple and pear fruits turn brown and black, respectively, shrivel, and remain attached to the spur and become mummified. The disease symptoms may advance downward from the blossoms, shoots, or fruit through the larger twigs and branches causing stem cankers.

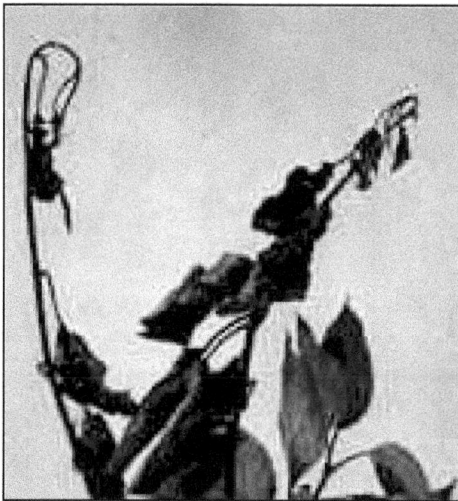

Figure 34: Fire Blight of Apple – Shepherds' Hook S.

Management

☆ Cultural practices like pruning of blighted twigs, branches and cankers reduce the inoculum spread.

☆ Insect vectors like aphids, ants, plant bugs and leaf hoppers should be controlled with proper insecticide application. Bordeaux mixture is also effective as blossom sprays.

☆ Use of resistant varieties like Red Delicious, North-west greening and Winesap.

Crown Gall of Apple

Causal Organism: *Agrobacterium tumefaciens*

Symptoms

In case of crown gall, globular, elongated or irregular galls are produced at or near the graft union. Galls vary in size from 0.6-10 cm in diameter and in extreme cases may go upto 0.3 m or more. In case of hairy root excessive fibrous roots originate from one place to give broom type appearance.

Management

☆ Good sanitation and cultural practices like discarding all symptomatic planting stock, budding rather than grafting and choosing resistant rootstocks minimizes disease.

☆ Dipping of seeds or root system of seedlings or rootstocks in *Agrobacterium radiobacter* – Strain K84 suspension controls effectively.

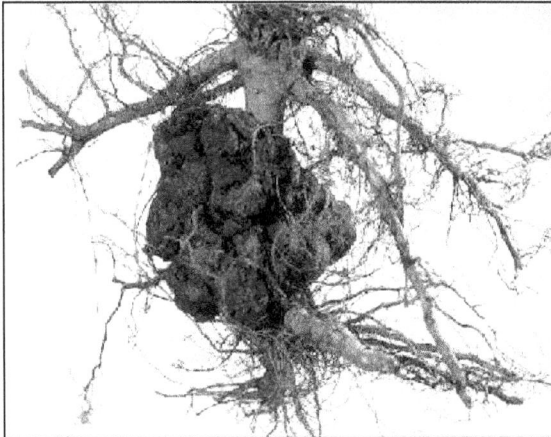

Figure 35: Crown Gall of Apple.

Wilt on Tomato

Causal Organism: *Pseudomonas solanacearum* (*Ralstonia solanacearum*)

Bacterial wilt caused by *R. solanacearum* affects more than 200 different plant species, including tomato, potato, brinjal, banana, geranium, ginger, tobacco, capsicums, olive and the flowering plant *Arabidopsis thaliana*. There is no cure.

Symptoms

Bacterial wilt on solanaceous crops appears as a sudden wilt. Infected young plants die rapidly, older plants first show wilting of the youngest leaves, or one-sided wilting and stunting, and finally the plants wilt permanently and die. In some plants, such as tomato, excessive adventitious roots may form. The vascular tissues of stems, roots, and tubers turn brown, and in cross sections they ooze a whitish bacterial exudates. Bacterial pockets develop around the vascular bundles in the pith and in the cortex, and roots and especially tubers often rot and disintegrate by the time the plant wilts permanently.

Management

☆ Cultivation of resistant varieties.

☆ Soil solarization with transparent polyethylene sheet for 8 to 10 weeks during March to June coupled with addition of antagonistic bacteria *Pseudomonas fluorescens* and *Bacillus* sp. favour multiplication of antagonistic bacteria and reduces the pathogen population.

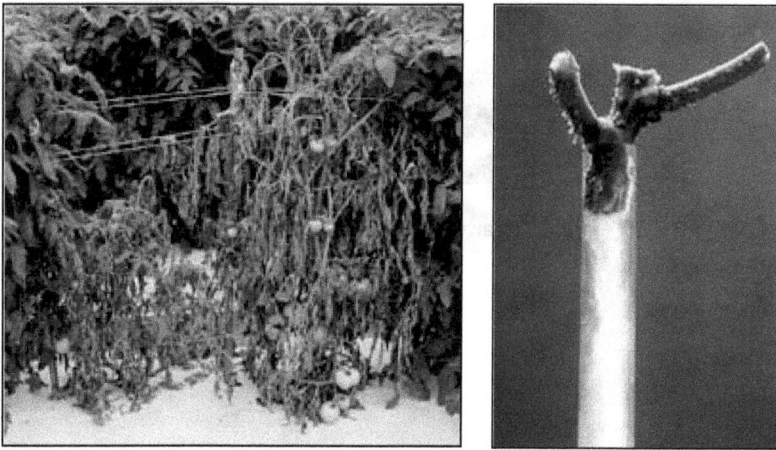

Figure 36: Tomato Wilt Caused by *Ralstonia solanacearum* Symptoms and Oozing of Bacterial Cells from Cut Ends into Water.

Common Scab of Potato

Causal Organism: *Streptomyces scabies*

Symptoms

The symptoms of common scab of potato appear on tubers as small brownish and slightly raised spots which later enlarge, coalesce and become corky. Multiple types of symptoms such as slight brownish roughening of tuber skin, proliferated lenticels with hard corky deposition, concentric series of wrinkled layers of cork around central black core, raised rough and corky pustules, and deep pits (3-4 mm) surrounded by hard corky tissue are produced.

Management

☆ Disease-free tubers should be used as seed.

☆ Delayed sowing escapes the diseases severity.

☆ Adaptation of crop rotation. Four years rotation with wheat-oat followed by potato-onion-maize is recommended.

☆ Maintenance of soil moisture up to the field capacity also reduces the disease.

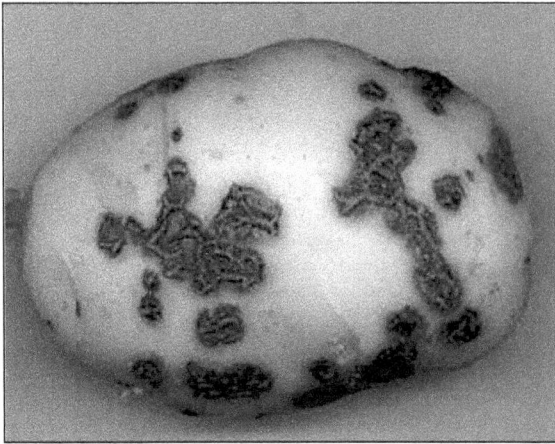

Figure 37: Potato Tuber with Symptoms of Common Scab.

7

Plant Viruses and Viroids

Viruses (Latin word for *'poison'*) are ultra-microscopic, obligate parasites containing nucleic acid and proteins that multiply only in living cells and has the ability to cause disease in plants, animals, fungi, bacteria and algae. There are over 2000 identified species of virus of which approximately 1000 species are phytopathogenic.

Virology: Study of viruses is called Virology.

Beijerinck, M.W.N [1898] is considered as father of virology, he made a detailed study of 'Tobacco mosaic disease' in plants and referred the causal agent as a **'virus'**.

Virus particles generally consist of infectious nucleic acid (DNA or RNA) encapsulated within the protein coat called **'capsid'**. Hence, the virus is referred as **'nucleocapsid'** and infectious virus particles as **'virions'**.

An incomplete virion without protein coat, *i.e.*, infective naked circular single stranded RNA (ribonucleic acid) capable of independent replication within a plant cell is termed as **'viroid'**.

Important Characteristics of Plant Viruses

- ☆ Ultra-microscopic.
- ☆ Highly intracellular with in the host cell in the presence of ribosomes (absolute parasites).
- ☆ Do not undergo binary fission, multiply only in terms of genetic material.
- ☆ Majority contains RNA.
- ☆ Obligate parasites.

☆ Do not have any enzyme system responsible for production of energy but have genetic information which commands the host cell to produce enzymes.

☆ Can pass through bacteria-proof filters.

☆ Have definite shapes that are spheres, rods or helical.

☆ Antigenic due to protein coat, so produces antibodies.

Often it is debated whether the viruses should be considered as living or non-living as they have the characteristics of both the groups. Viruses are infectious agents with both living and non-living characteristics.

1. Living characteristics of viruses:

   a. They reproduce at a fantastic rate, but only in living host cells.

   b. They can mutate.

2. Nonliving characteristics of viruses:

   a. They are acellular, that is, they contain no cytoplasm or cellular organelles.

   b. They carry out no metabolism on their own and must replicate using the host cell's metabolic machinery. In other words, viruses don't grow and divide. Instead, new viral components are synthesized and assembled within the infected host cell.

   c. The vast majority of viruses possess either DNA or RNA but not both.

Plant Virus Shapes and Sizes

The plant viruses exist in different shapes and sizes. Viruses are usually much smaller than bacteria and are submicroscopic. Most viruses range in size from 5 to 300 nanometers (nm), although some can be up to 2,000 nm long (1 nm=10^{-9} m). The shapes of plant viruses also vary from small spherical (icosahedral) (Cucumber mosaic virus - 29 nm dia.) shape to bullet-shaped (Bacilliform) (Potato yellow dwarf *nucleorhabdovirus* – 75x380 nm) to rod-shaped (Tobacco mosaic *tobamovirus* – 18x300 nm) to short flexuous rods (Potato virus X *potexvirus* – 13x515 nm) to medium flexous rods (Potato virus Y *potyvirus* – 11x730 nm) to long flexuous rods (Citrus tristeza *closterovirus* - 15x2000 nm).

Transmission of Plant Viruses

Plant viruses rarely come out of the plant spontaneously. Therefore, viruses are not disseminated by wind or water. Even when they are carried in debris or plant sap, they would cause infections only when they come in contact with the contents of wounded live cell. Viruses are transmitted from plant to plant in a number of ways *viz.*, vegetative propagation, mechanical transmission through sap, and by seed, pollen, insects, mites, nematodes, fungi, dodder etc.

1. **Vegetative propagation:** Any part of plant used for vegetative propagation can carry the viruses to the progeny. Thus viruses are transmitted by budding, grafting, cuttings, tubers, corms, bulbs, rhizomes etc. This

mode of transmission is most important for ornamental trees and shrubs propagated by any such means and the field crops like potato and most florists' crops that are usually propagated by tubers, corms or cuttings. In trees, particularly, viruses are transmitted through natural root grafts of adjacent infected plants. For several tree viruses, natural grafts and dodders are the only known means of tree-to-tree spread of the virus. Banana bunchy top *nanavirus* is transmitted through suckers.

2. **Mechanical transmission through sap:** Under natural conditions, direct transfer of sap through contact of one plant with another is uncommon. Such mechanical transmission may take place between closely placed plants. Strong wind may cause the leaves of adjacent plants to rub together, and if wounded, some of their sap is exchanged, thus transmitting any virus present in the sap. Potato Virus X (PVX) and Tobacco Mosaic Virus (TMV) are most easily transmitted in this way.

   Plants are wounded by man during cultural practices in field or greenhouse, and some of the virus-infected sap adhering to tools, hands or clothes is accidentally transferred to wounded plants. TMV on tobacco and tomato spreads rapidly in this way. Occasionally virus-infected sap is transferred from one plant to another on the mouthparts or body of animals feeding on and moving among the plants. Mechanical transmission is one of the most authentic means to prove the ability of infection by a virus.

3. **Seed transmission:** This is not as common as the above two methods. More than 100 viruses are reported to be transmitted by seed. However, only a small portion (1-30 per cent) of the seeds derived from virus-infected plants transmit the virus. In some cases as Tobacco Ring Spot Virus (TRSV) in soybean, almost 100 per cent of seeds of infected plants can transmit the virus to the seedlings grown from them. Barley Stripe Mosaic Virus also has high seed transmission rate of 50-100 per cent. In most cases, the virus comes primarily through the ovule of infected plants. Prunus necrotic ringspot *ilarvirus* is seed transmitted in *Prunus pennsylvanica* up to 80 per cent.

4. **Pollen transmission:** Virus transmitted by pollen not only infects the seed and the seedling growing from it, but more importantly it can also spread through fertilized flower and down into the mother plant, that thus becomes infected with the virus. This method is important in stone fruit ring spot virus of some plants. Prunus necrotic ringspot *ilarvirus* is transmitted by pollen to the seed and also to the pollinated plant.

5. **Mite transmission:** Members of the family Eriophyidae are shown to transmit nine viruses, including Wheat Streak Mosaic, Pigeon Pea Sterility Mosaic, Peach Mosaic and Fig Mosaic viruses. These mites have piercing and sucking mouthparts. Mite transmission appears to be specific, since each of the mite species has a restricted host range. In such cases a particular mite is the only known vector for the virus or viruses transmitted by it. Some of mite-transmitted viruses are non-circulatory

(stylet-borne), whereas others are circulatory. Onion mite-borne latent *potexvirus* is transmitted by *Aceria tulipae* (Eriophyidae).

6. **Nematode transmission:** About 12 viruses are shown to be transmitted by one or more species of three genera of soil inhabiting, ectoparasitic nematodes. Members of the genera *Longidorus* and *Xiphinema* are vectors of Tobacco Ring Spot Virus, Tomato Ring Spot Virus, Raspberry Ring Spot Virus, Cherry Leaf Roll Virus, Tomato Black Ring Virus, Grapevine Fan-leaf Virus etc., whereas those of the genus *Trichodorus* transmit Tobacco Rattle Virus and Pea Early Browning Virus. Nematodes feed on roots of infected plant and then move on to roots of healthy plants. Larvae as well as adults can acquire and transmit the viruses.

7. **Fungal transmission:** *Olpidium*, a root-infecting chytrid, is known to transmit at least four viruses *viz.*, Tobacco Necrosis Virus, Cucumber Necrosis Virus, Lettuce Big Vein Virus and Tobacco Stunt Virus. Four other fungi, *Synchytrium, Polymyxa, Spongospora* and *Pythium* transmit Potato Virus X, Wheat Mosaic Virus, Potato Mop Top Virus and Beet Necrotic Yellow Vein Virus, respectively. The viruses are carried in or on the zoospores and resting spores.

8. **Dodder transmission:** Several viruses can spread through the bridge formed between infected and healthy plants by twining stems dodder (*Cuscuta* sp), a parasitic phanerogam. Many viruses spread in this way between plants of widely different taxonomic species. Ex. *Cuscuta subinclusa* and *C. reflexa* were able to transmit tristeza, sporosis and vein enation viruses of citrus.

9. **Insect transmission:** The most common and economically important method of transmission of viruses in the field is by insects. The order Homoptera, which includes the most potential virus vector groups such as aphids and leafhoppers, contains the largest number and the most important insect vectors of plant viruses. White flies, mealy bugs, scale insects and plant hoppers belonging to this order also transmit viruses but are not economically as important as aphids and leafhoppers. Other insect vectors are true bugs (Hemiptera), thrips (Thysanoptera), beetles (Coleoptera) and the grasshoppers (Orthoptera). The most important vector groups *viz.*, aphids, leafhoppers and other members of Homoptera, as well as true bugs, have piercing and sucking mouthparts; all other vectors have chewing mouthparts and the transmission by the latter is much less common.

On the basis of virus-vector relationship with aphid vectors (where virus is carried by vector; and behaviour of virus within the vector), the viruses are categorized as follows:

(a) **Non-circulative:** These are the viruses which do not circulate in the insect body from the mouthparts to the salivary glands but are carried on their stylets (sucking mouthparts). The infectivity (viruliferous nature of the vector) is lost during molting process. In this category there are two types:

i) **Non-persistent**: The vectors can transmit the virus immediately after acquiring the virus and the ability to transmit the virus is lost within a few minutes to few hours (usually within 4 hours) after the acquisition. The viruses are mostly limited to the stylet only and are lost by moulting. Hence they are also called 'stylet-borne viruses'. Most mosaic viruses are transmitted this way. Ex: Bean yellow mosaic *potyvirus* in aphid, *Acyrthosiphon pisum*.

ii) **Semi-persistent**: The vectors can transmit the virus after a few minutes after acquisition and the ability to transmit the virus is lost after 3 to 4 days of acquisition. These viruses are retained only up to foregut of the vector and never enter the midgut region and may or may not be lost by moulting. Ex: Beet yellows *closterovirus* in aphid, *Myzus persicae*.

(b) **Circulative:** These viruses get circulated in the insect body, *i.e.*, enter the midgut after acquisition and pass through the midgut wall to the haemolymph and reach the salivary glands from where the virus is reintroduced into healthy plant through the stylets. The viruliferous nature of the vector is retained even after molting process. Under this category two types exist.

i) **Non-propagative**: The virus particles pass through the midgut wall to the salivary glands without any multiplication. This is evident as there is no increase in the number of particles acquired by the vector in its body till final transmission of these particles, as the ability to transmit the virus is lost within a few days and is not lost by moulting. Ex: Bhendi yellow vein mosaic *bigeminivirus* in white fly, *Bemisia tabaci*.

ii) **Propagative:** These are some of the circulative viruses that may multiply in their vectors. This is evident as the number of particles increase in the insect body, since their entry till their transmission, as the ability to transmit the virus after single acquisition is retained throughout the remaining life of the insect and not lost by moulting. In some cases, the virus is retained trans-ovarially during next one or few generations. Ex. Potato yellow dwarf *Nucleorhabdovirus* in the leafhopper vector, *Agallia constricta*.

The viruses transmitted by insects with chewing mouthparts may also be non-circulative or circulative.

Aphids are the most important insect vectors of plant viruses and transmit the great majority of all stylet-borne viruses. More than 200 species are known as vectors of plant viruses. As a rule several aphid species can transmit the same stylet-borne virus and the same aphid species can transmit several viruses, but in many cases, the vector-virus relationship is quite specific. Aphids generally acquire the stylet-borne virus after a brief feeding period (lasting for 30 seconds or less) on the diseased plant, and can transmit the virus immediately after transfer to and feeding on a healthy plant for a similar brief period. After acquisition, the aphids remain viruliferous for a few minutes to several hours, after which they can no longer transmit the virus. In some cases of aphid transmission of circulative viruses, aphids can not transmit the virus immediately but must wait several hours after the feeding. However, once they start to transmit the virus, they continue to do so for many days. The stylet-borne viruses are carried on the tips of the stylets. Several species of leafhoppers are involved in transmission of a number of plant viruses. Leafhopper transmitted viruses cause disturbance primarily in the phloem region. All leafhopper transmitted viruses are circulative and several are known to multiply in the vector *i.e.*, propagative. Most of the leafhoppers require a feeding period of one to several days before they become viruliferous, but once they acquire the virus they remain viruliferous for the rest of their lives.

Classification of Plant Viruses

In the 6th report of the International Committee on Taxonomy of Viruses (ICTV), plant viruses were classified into genera and families. The 7th report of the ICTV listed a total of 904 plant viruses classified as members or tentative members of 70 genera based on the structure of the genome *i.e.*, nucleic acid. The plant viruses vary very much in the nature of the genome they carry. It ranges from a simple positive single stranded RNA to double stranded DNA *i.e.*, 1) ss RNA a) Positive [+ve] sense i) Monopartite, ii) Bipartite, iii) Tripartite, iv) Multipartite; b) Negative [-ve] sense RNA; 2) ds RNA; 3) ss DNA; 4) ds DNA. The classification also considered the presence or absence of lipoprotein envelope covering on the nucleocapsid.

Partial list of viruses, infecting horticultural crops, named in alphabetical order and their abbreviations as used in the 7th ICTV report, which has recently been published, are furnished here.

A. Genome dsDNA (Not-enveloped)

1. Family: Caulimoviridae

Genera	Type Species	Vector
Caulimovirus	Cauliflower mosaic virus (CaMV)	Aphids, Myzus persicae
Badnavirus	Cocoa swollen shoot Virus	Mealy bugs Planococcoides njalensis

B. Genome ssDNA (Not-enveloped)

1. Family: Geminiviridae

Genera	Type Species	Vector
Curtovirus	Beet curly top virus	Leafhoppers, Circulifer tenellus
Begomovirus	Bean golden mosaic virus	Whiteflies, Bemesia tabaci
Topocuvirus	Tomato pseudo-curly top virus	Tree hoppers, Micrutalis malleifera

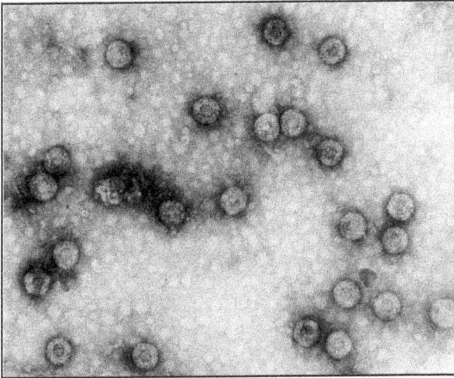

Figure 38: Cauliflower Mosaic
caulimovirus.

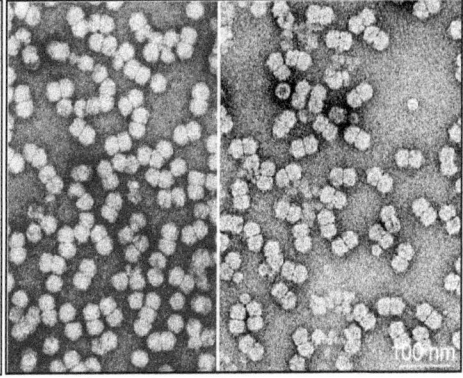

Figure 39: Bean Golden Mosaic
begomovirus.

C. Genome dsRNA

1. Family: Reoviridae

Genera	Type Species	Vector
Phytoreovirus	Wound tumor virus	Leafhopper, *Agallia constricta*

2. Family: Not assigned (dsRNA) (Bipartite) (Not-enveloped)

Genera	Type Species	Vector
Varicosavirus	Lettuce big-vein virus (LBVV)	Fungus, *Olpidium brassicae*

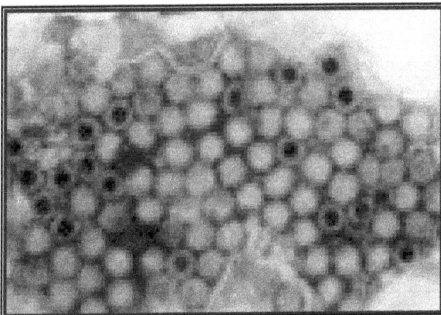

Figure 40: Wound Tumor *phytoreovirus.*

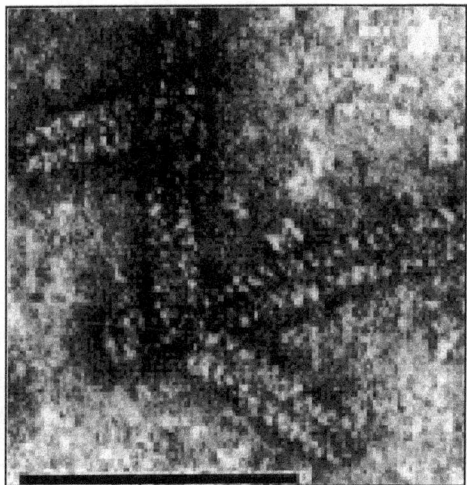

Figure 41: *Varicosavirus.*

Genome (-ve) ssRNA (Enveloped)

1. Family: Rhabdoviridae

Genera	Type Species	Vector
Cytothabdovirus	Lettuce necrotic yellow virus (LNYV)	Aphids, *Hyperomyzus lactucae*
Nucleorhabdovirus	Potato yellow dwarf virus (PYDV)	Leafhopper, *Agallia constricta*

2. Family: Bunyaviridae

Genera	Type Species	Vector
Tospovirus	Tomato Spotted Wilt Virus (TSWV)	Thrips, *Thrips tabaci*
Ophio virus	Citrus sporosis virus (CSV)	No vector

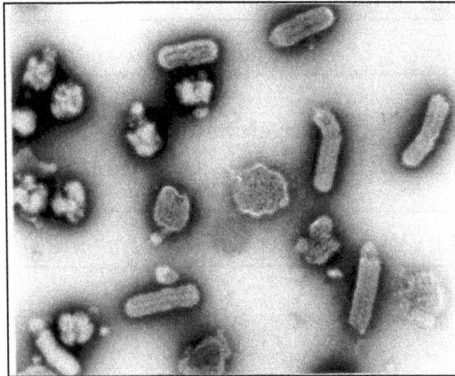

Figure 42: *Nucleorhabdovirus.*

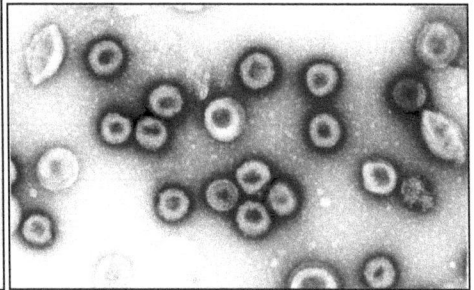

Figure 43: Tomato Spotted Wilt *tospovirus.*

Genome (+) ssRNA (Tripartite) (Not-enveloped)

1. Family: Bromoviridae

Genera	Type Species	Vector
Cucumo virus	Cucumber mosaic virus (CMV)	Aphids, *Aphis craccivora* and *Myzus persicae*
Ilavirus	Prunus necrotic ring spot virus (PNRSV)	No vector

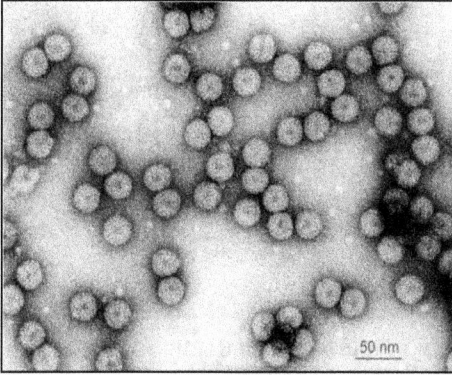

Figure 44: Cucumber Mosaic
cucumovirus.

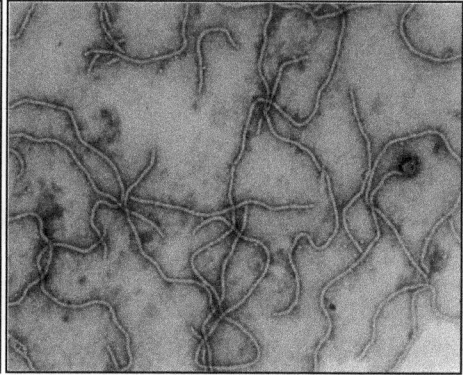

Figure 45: Beet Yellows *closterovirus.*

2. Family: Closteroviridae (Monopartite) (Not-enveloped)

Genera	Type Species	Vector
Closterovirus	Beet yellows virus (BYV)	Aphids, Myzus persicae and Aphis fabae
Crinivirus	Lettuce infectious yellows virus (LIYV)	Whiteflies, Bemesia tabaci
Ampelovirus	Grapevine leafroll-associated virus 3	Mealy bugs, Pseudococcus longispinus

3. Family: Comoviridae (Bi-partite) (Not-enveloped)

Genera	Type Species	Vector
Comovirus	Cowpea mosaic virus	Beetles; Acalymma vittatum
Nepovirus	Tobacco ring spot virus (TRSV)	Nematodes, Longidorus elongatus
Fabavirus	Broad bean wilt virus-1 (BBWV-1)	Aphids, Acyrthosiphon pisum

3. Family: Luteoviridae (Mono- or bipartite) (Not-enveloped)

Genera	Type Species	Vector
Polero virus	Potato leaf roll virus (PLRV)	Aphids, Myzus persicae
Enamovirus	Pea enation mosaic virus -1 (PEMV-1)	Aphids, Acyrthosiphon pisum

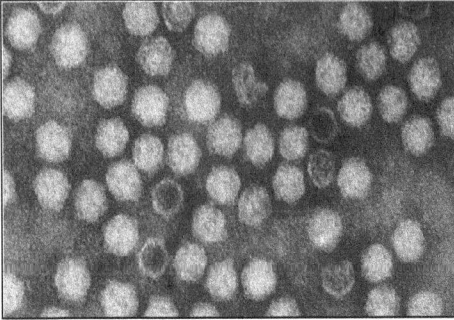

Figure 46: Cowpea Mosaic *comovirus*.

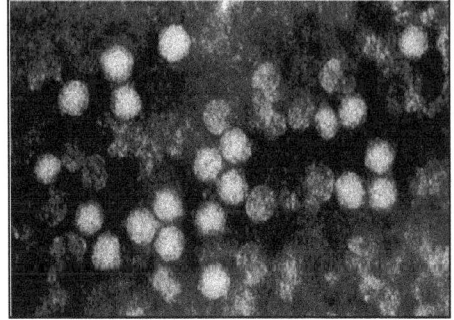

Figure 47: Pea Enation Mosaic *enamovirus*.

5. Family: Potyviridae (Mono-partite) (Not-enveloped)

Genera	Type Species	Vector
Potyvirus	Potato Virus-Y (PVY)	Aphids, Myzus persicae
Ipomovirus	Sweet potato mild mosaic virus (SPMMV)	Whitefly, Bemisia tabaci

6. Family: Sequiviridae (Mono-partite) (Not-enveloped)

Genera	Type Species	Vector
Sequivirus	Parsnip yellow fleck virus	Aphids, Cavariella aegopodii
Waikavirus	Rice tungro spherical virus (RTSV)	Leafhoppers, Nephotettix virescens

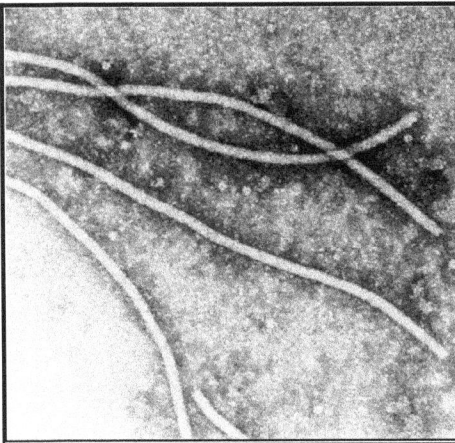

Figure 48: Potato Virus Y *potyvirus*.

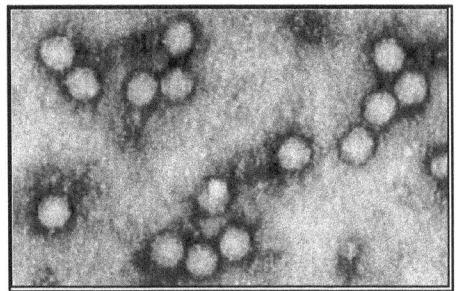

Figure 49: Rice Tungro Spherical *waikavirus*.

7. Family: Tombusviridae (Mono- or bi-partite) (Not-enveloped)

Genera	Type Species	Vector
Tombusvirus	Tomato bushy stunt virus (TBSV)	No vector
Carmovirus	Carnation mottle virus (CarMV)	No vector
Necrovirus	Tobacco necrosis virus-A (TNV-A)	Fungus, *Olpidium brassicae*
Dianthovirus	Carnation ring spot virus (CRSV)	Nematode, *Longidorus elongatus*

8. Family: Flexiviridae (+ve) (ssRNA) (Mono-partite) (Not-enveloped)

Genera	Type Species	Vector
Potex virus	Potato virus X(PVX)	No vector
Carlavirus	Carnation latent virus (CLV)	Aphids, *Myzus persicae*
Foveavirus	Apple stem pitting virus (ASPV)	No Vector
Allexivirus	Shallot virus X (Sh VX)	No vector
Capillovirus	Apple stem grooving virus (ASGV)	No Vector
Trichovirus	Apple chlorotic leaf spot virus (ACLSV)	No Vector
Vitivirus	Grapevine virus A (GVA)	Mealy bugs, *Pseudococcus longispinus*

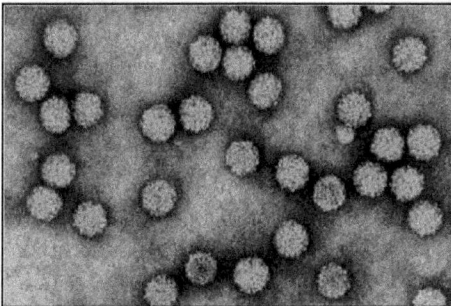

Figure 50: Tomato Bushy Stunt *tombusvirus*.

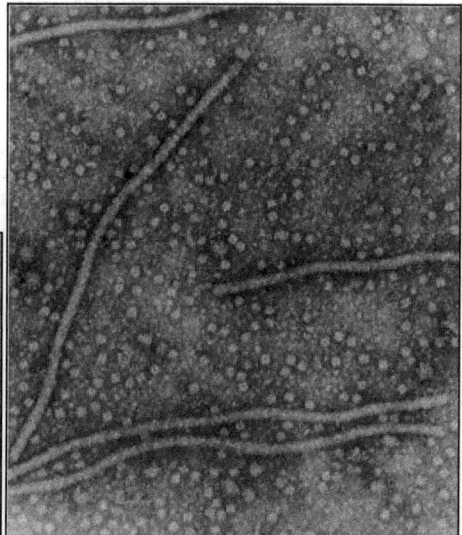

Figure 51: Potato Virus X *potexvirus*.

9. Family: Tymoviridae (+ve) (ssRNA) (Mono-partite) (Not-enveloped)

Genera	Type Species	Vector
Tymovirus	Turnip yellow mosaic virus (TYMV)	Flea beetles, *Phyllotreta* spp.
Maculavirus	Grapevine fleck virus (GFkV)	No vector

10. Unassigned (+ve) (ssRNA) (Bi-partite) (Not-enveloped)

Genera	Type Species	Vector
Tobravirus	Tobacco rattle virus (TRV)	Paratrichodorus allius

11. Unassigned (+ve) (ss RNA) (Mono-partite) (Not-enveloped)

Genera	Type Species	Vector
Tobamovirus	Tobacco mosaic virus (TMV)	No vector

12. Unassigned (+ve) (ssRNA) (Mono-partite) (Not-enveloped)

Genera	Type Species	Vector
Pomovirus	Potato mop-top virus (PMTV)	Fungus, Spongospora subterranea

13. Unassigned (+ve) (ssRNA)(Multi-partite) (Not-enveloped)

Genera	Type Species	Vector
Benyvirus	Beet necrotic yellow vein virus (BNYVV)	Fungus, Polymyxa betae

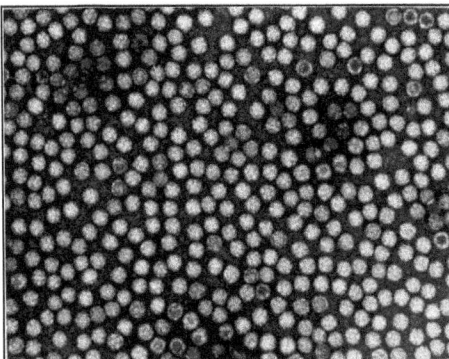

Figure 52: Turnip Yellow Mosaic *tymovirus.*

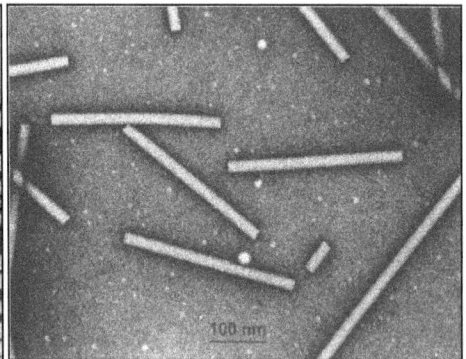

Figure 53: Tobacco Mosaic *tobamovirus.*

14. Unassigned (+ve) (ssRNA) (Mono-partite) (Not-enveloped)

Genera	Type Species	Vector
Sobemo virus	Southern bean mosaic virus (SBMV)	Beetles, *Ceratoma trifurcata*

15. Unassigned (+ve) (ssRNA) (No true particles)

Genera	Type Species	Vector
Umbravirus	Carrot mottle virus (CMoV)	Aphids, *Cavariella aegopodii*

16. Unassigned (+ve) (ssRNA) (Mono-partite) (Not-enveloped)

Genera	Type Species	Vector
Idaeovirus	Raspberry bushy dwarf virus (RBDV)	No Vector

Symptoms Caused by Plant Viruses

Viruses cause several kinds of symptoms in diseased plants. The viruses may be **systemic** *i.e.*, associated with each stage of plant growth; or **localized** *i.e.*, being restricted to some parts of plant only. In almost all viral diseases occurring in the field, the virus is present throughout the plant (systemic infection) and the symptoms are called systemic symptoms. In many artificially inoculated plants and in some natural infections, viruses form local lesions (local infection).

The most common and sometimes the only kind of symptom is reduced growth rate the plant. This results into various degrees of dwarfing or stunting of the entire plant. All viral diseases cause some degree of reduction in total yield.

The most obvious symptoms are usually those appearing on the leaf, but some viruses may cause striking symptoms on the stem, roots and fruit with or without symptom development on the leaves. Many viruses may infect some hosts without causing development of visible symptoms. Such viruses are called **latent viruses** and the hosts are called **symptomless carriers.** In some cases with plants which remain symptom-less temporarily but under certain environmental conditions like high or low temperatures, they develop symptoms. Such symptoms are called **masked.** Finally, plants may show acute or severe symptoms soon as the environmental conditions help in the symptom development.

The most common types of plant symptoms produced by systemic virus infections are **mosaics** and **ring spots.** A large number of other less common symptoms are stunt, dwarf, leaf roll, yellows, streak, pox, enation, tumors, pitting of stem, pitting of fruit, flattening and distortion of stem etc. These symptoms may be accompanied by other symptoms on other parts of the same plant.

1. Mosaics

These are characterized by light-green, yellow, or white areas intermingled with the normal green colour of the leaves or fruit; or whitish area intermingled with areas of the normal colour of flower or fruit. Depending on the intensity or pattern of discolorations, mosaic-type symptoms may be described as mottling, streak, ring pattern, line pattern, vein-clearing, vein-banding, vein-thickening, chlorotic spotting etc. Ex: Tomato Mosaic *tobamovirus*.

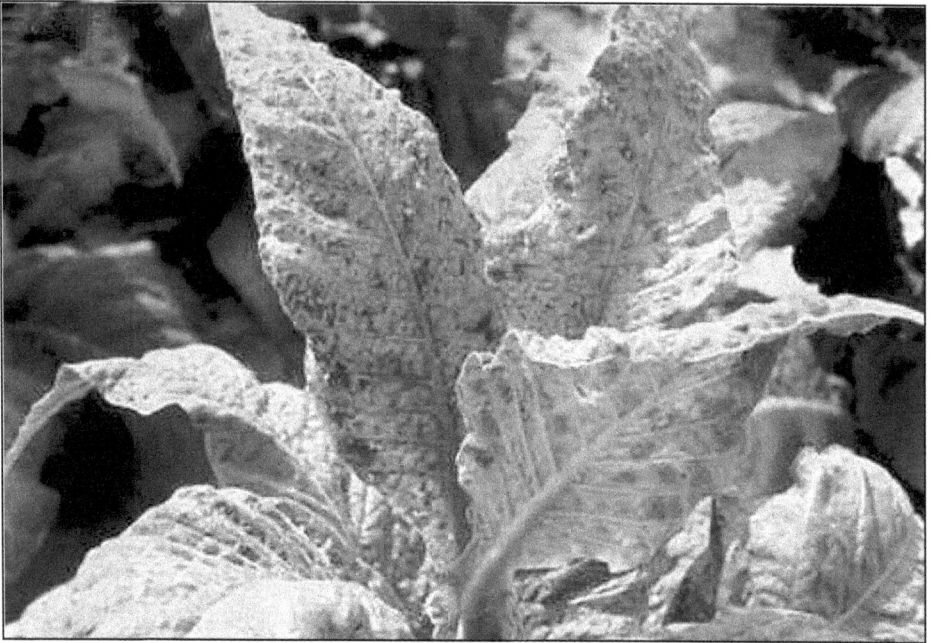

Figure 54: Mosaic Symptoms on Tobacco Caused by Tobacco Mosaic *tobamovirus*.

2. Mottles

It is a kind of mosaic, where irregular patterns of indistinct light and dark areas develop on the leaves. Like mosaics, there are green and white or green and yellow areas. Ex: Cucumber Green Mild Mottle mosaic *tobamovirus*.

3. Yellows (Chlorosis)

In extreme cases of mosaics and mottles the leaf may become almost completely yellow due to chlorosis. This symptom is also common in phytoplasma diseases. Ex: Beet Yellows *closterovirus*; Aster Yellows (Phytoplasma).

4. Vein-clearing

In this case, chlorosis of leaf tissue occurs in close proximity of the veins. The tissue close to veins turns yellow and the remaining area appears green. Ex: Bhendi Yellow Vein Mosaic *begomovirus*.

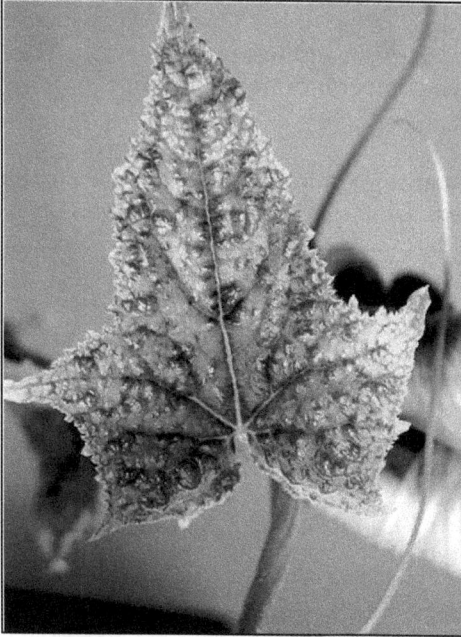

Figure 55: Mottle Symptoms on Cucurbits Caused by Cucumber Green Mild Mottle Mosaic *tobamovirus.*

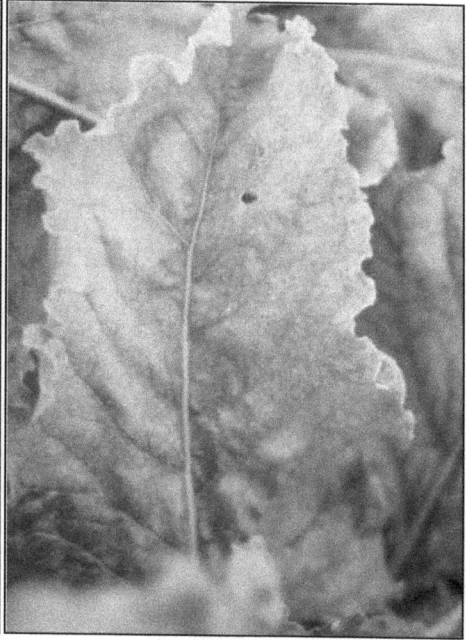

Figure 56: Chlorosis of Beet Caused by Beet Yellows *closterovirus.*

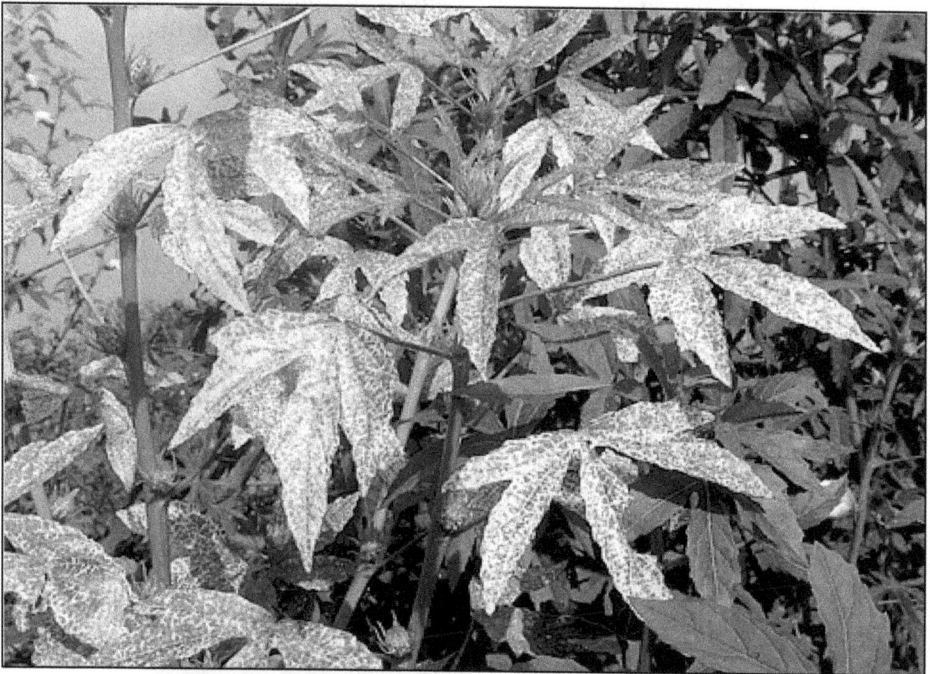

Figure 57: Vein-clearing Symptom in Bhendi Caused by Bhendi Yellow Vein Mosaic *begomovirus.*

5. Vein-banding

Here the parenchyma close to the veins is green and rest of the lamina surface shows chlorosis, *i.e.*, becomes yellow. Ex: Cucumber mosaic *cucumovirus*.

6. Ring Spots

These are characterized by the appearance of chlorotic or necrotic rings on leaves and sometimes also on fruit and stem. Ex: Papaya Ring Spot *potyvirus*.

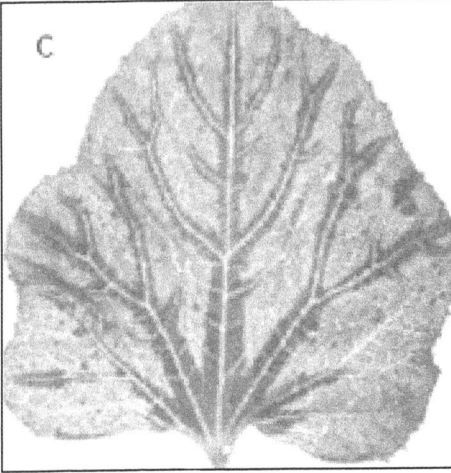

Figure 58: Vein-banding in Cucurbits Due to Infection by Cucumber Mosaic *cucumovirus*.

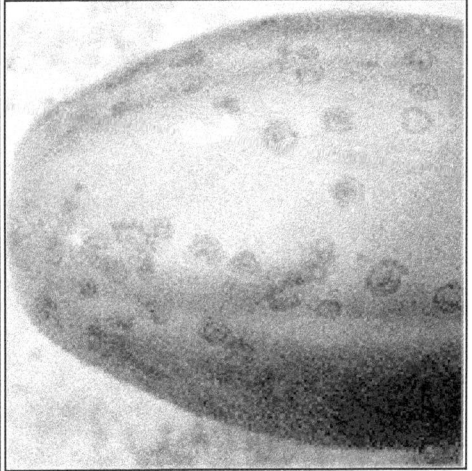

Figure 59: Ring Spots on Papaya Fruits Caused by Papaya Ring Spot *potyvirus*.

7. Enations

These are small outgrowths on leaf, stem etc. This is usually associated with mosaics. Ex: Pea Enation Mosaic *umbravirus*.

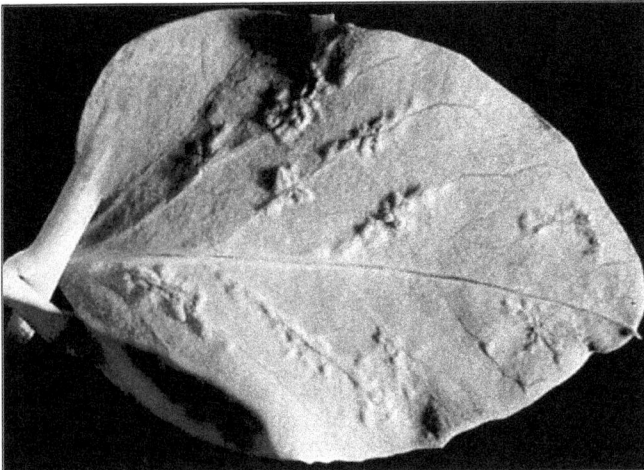

Figure 60: Enations on Pea Leaf Due to Pea Enation Mosaic *umbravirus*.

8. Leaf-curling or Leaf-rolling

These are common in papaya, tomato, potato etc., where leaves become curled and rolled to varying extents. Ex: Potato leaf roll *polerovirus*.

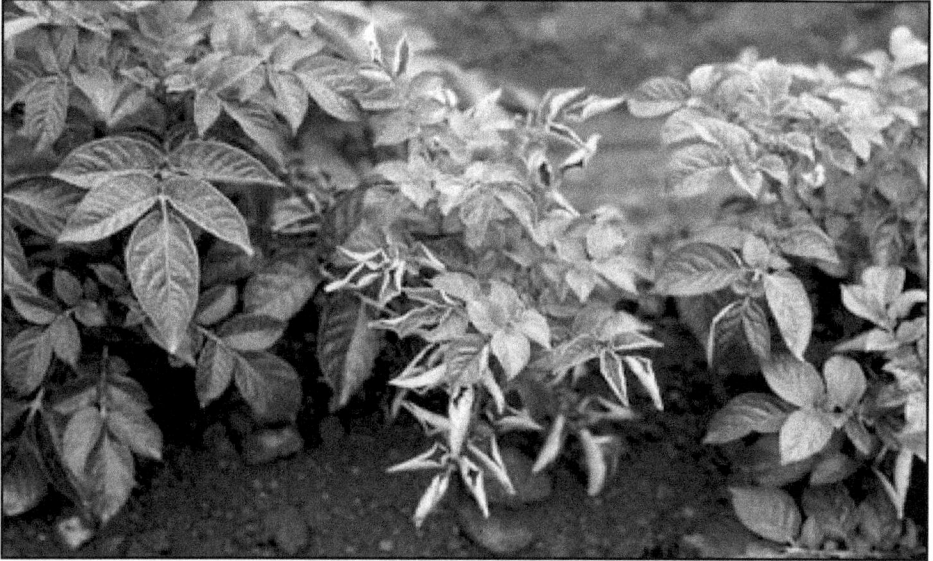

Figure 61: Potato Leaves Showing Leaf Roll on Infection with Potato Leaf Roll *polerovirus*.

9. Fern-leaf, Shoe String

Here leaf lamina is greatly suppressed. Ex: Papaya Mosaic.

10. Stunting

The general growth of entire plant is affected resulting into unusually shorter size of plant. Ex: *Chrysanthemum* Stunt (Figure 63).

11. Virescence

Here entire flower or petals turn to green colour. It is a type of phyllody. This symptom is common in phytoplasma diseases.

12. Tumors

These are gall-like structures developing on roots or stems. In Fiji disease of sugarcane, elongated galls on leaf are formed. Ex: Wound Tumor Virus *Phytoreovirus*.

13. Witches' Broom

The leaves become very much reduced with shortened inter-nodes. There is abnormal growth of clustering leaves turning into a densely-packed broom-like structure. This symptom is common in phytoplasma diseases. Ex: Potato Witches' broom.

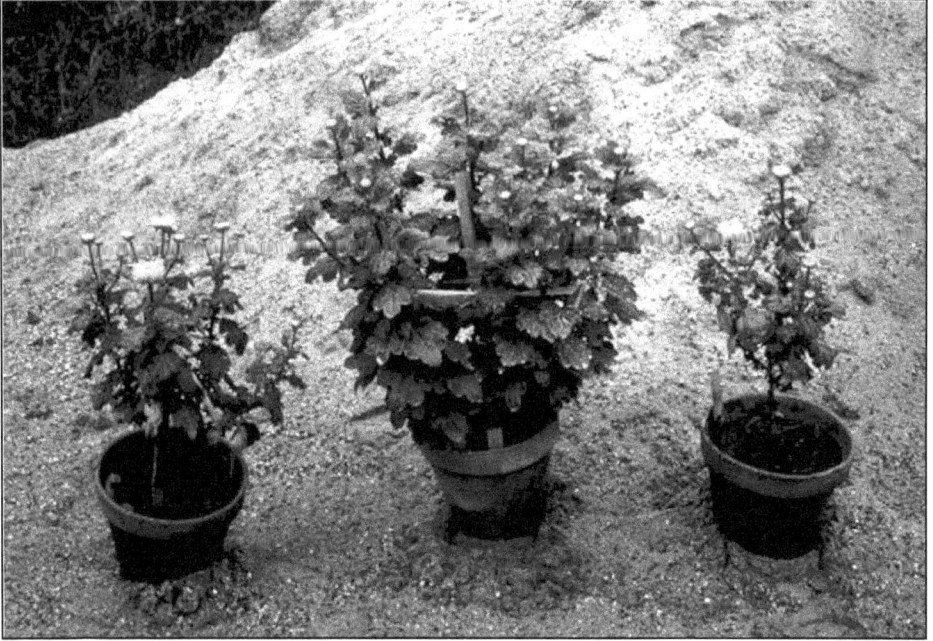

Figure 62: Chrysanthemum Stunt Viroid Infected Plants on either Side of Healthy Plant.

14. Little Leaf

The leaves are reduced in size and the lamina is very much suppressed. This symptom is common in phytoplasma diseases. Ex: Brinjal Little Leaf (*Phytoplasma*).

Important Diseases Caused by Plant Viruses

1. Tomato Mosaic Disease

The disease is caused by Tomato mosaic *tobamovirus*.

This disease is widespread in distribution and is known to occur wherever tomato is grown. The disease reduces plant vigor and yield by 3 to 25 per cent.

Symptoms: 1) Appearance of pale and dark green mosaic pattern on the leaves of infected plant. 2) Young leaves are malformed; some times stunted and

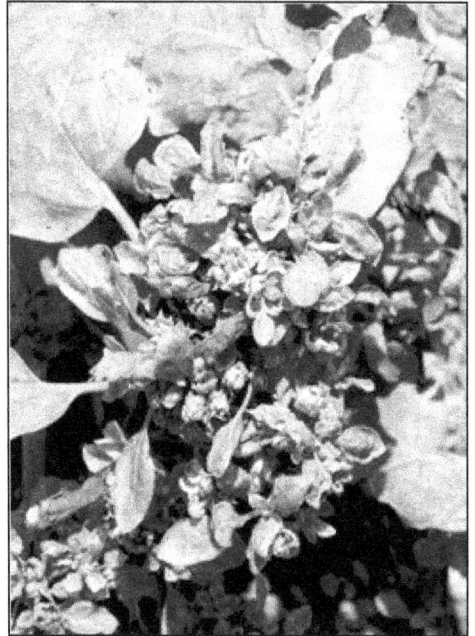

Figure 63: Brinjal Little Leaf Caused by *phytoplasma.*

may become fern-shaped. 3) Necrosis of leaves, stems, petiole and some times fruits may be seen. 4) Necrosis is more severe in mixed infection. 5) Infected plants may remain stunted.

Transmission

Infected seeds and plants are important sources of inoculum in nature. Infected seeds usually transmit the virus year after year ensuring a permanent disease cycle. Further spread of disease takes place through mechanical means especially during transplanting by handling and other cultural operations.

Management

(1) Clean and healthy seed should be sown. Before sowing, seeds should be disinfected by soaking in 10 per cent (w/v) trisodium phosphate (Na_3PO_4) solution for 20 minutes to eliminate external seed infections. (2) Management of the disease through cross protection. (3) Use of resistant/tolerant cultivars should be preferred for economic management of the disease.

2. Yellow Vein Mosaic Disease of Okra

The disease is caused by Yellow vein mosaic virus *begomovirus*.

The virus is not sap transmissible but under artificial conditions, it could be transmitted by grafting.

Okra, usually called as Bhindi in Hindi, suffers from yellow vein mosaic disease which is much destructive in India, Pakistan and Bangladesh. This disease was first reported by Kulkarni during 1924 and has been studied in detail by different workers. The extent of loss due to this disease has been estimated to be as high as 85 to 96 per cent when the crop was found infected during early stage of growth.

Symptoms

(1) Vein-clearing and veinal chlorosis of leaves of infected plants are the most distinguishing characteristics of the disease. (2) Yellow network of veins is very conspicuous along with thickening of veins and veinlets. (3) In case of severe infection, chlorosis may extend to the inter-veinal areas, resulting in complete yellowing of leaves. (4) Fruits if develop, they are smaller in size, yellowish-green in colour and are malformed in appearance.

Host Range

Several weed hosts and roadside plants including *Croton sparsiflora, Malvastrum tricuspidatum* and *Ageratum* spp. are known to harbour the virus assisting in its perpetuation.

Transmission

The virus is transmitted by white fly, *Bemisia tabaci*.

Management

(1) Spray suitable insecticide starting from the 7-10 days of germination so as to manage insect vectors. Sprayings (4 to 6) of the mixture of dimecron and nuvan

@ 1 ml each, *i.e.*, 2 ml/3 liters of water should be done at 15 days intervals. Other insecticide like metasystox or rogor can also be used. (2) Destruction of weed and wild hosts should be done so as to avoid perpetuation of the virus. (3) Use of resistant/tolerant cultivars is recommended for the management of the disease in large scale cultivation.

3. Tobacco Mosaic Disease

The disease is caused by Tobacco mosaic *tobamovirus*.

The disease is widespread in occurrence and is well-known in all countries where tobacco is grown. As high as 55 per cent reduction in produce has been observed in different countries. The quality of the produce is also reduced considerably making it sub-standard in the market.

Symptoms

(1) Leaves of infected plants show mild clearing of veins. (2) Clearly visible mottle and mosaic occur in younger leaves later in the season. (3) Golden yellow mosaic or light green spots are seen on *Nicotiana sylvestris* cv. *Otlja* and tissue necrosis occurs within these spots in some other cultivars. (4) Wrinkling, crinkling, twisting of margins and narrowing of leaflets are also observed. (5) There are marked reduction in growth and substantial reduction in yield.

Host Range

The virus is preserved in nature in herbaceous and woody plants. Vegetables including tomato, potato and pepper grown indoors usually transmit the virus from crop to crop. The virus has wide host range and more than 550 species of flowering plants including 60 natural and many other experimental hosts are known. Natural hosts include several species of tobacco, tomato, potato, wild apple, plum and grapevine. Some strains of TMV also infect fungal species like *Erysiphe gramints*, *E. polygoni, Phyllactinia corylea* and *Sphacrotheca lanestris* and many other species.

Transmission

The virus may remain infective in the roots or organic matter of the soil for more than 2 years if such soil is not exposed to freezing and drying. The virus is easily transmitted by smoke through contact with susceptible plants. Mechanical transmission of TMV is unique among viruses. Weeding, uprooting, transplanting, inflorescence cutting and periodical harvesting usually create environment for the transmission of the virus from the source to the healthy plants. No insect vector is possibly known to exist; however, grass hoppers, butterfly and caterpillars are known to transmit the virus through mechanical means by contact.

Management

Experimental results have suggested some preventive measures *viz.*, 1) For seedling production, planting of only clean and healthy seed, free of plant-residues, should be done. 2) Use uncontaminated soils for seed production. 3) Disinfect all soils of unknown origin prior to sowing and produce only tobacco seedlings in flower beds. Do not use same flower beds for tomato and pepper seedlings.

4) All workers should disinfect their hands at regular intervals. Restrict smoking by workers. 5) All infected and suspected plants should be removed from the vicinity of the nurseries. 6) Grow tobacco in three-year crop rotation with maize and wheat, avoiding tomato and pepper crops. 7) Infection by mechanical inoculation can be reduced in limited area by spraying plants with skim milk or butter-milk. Leaves from healthy plants should be harvested first and then those from infected plants.

4. Bean Common Mosaic Disease

The disease is caused by Bean common mosaic *potyvirus*.

This disease is one of the most damaging diseases of this crop. High losses in bean yields have been observed when crop densities favour the occurrence and spread of natural infections.

Symptoms

(1) Mild to severe mosaic, vein-banding, leaf malformation and curling of leaves are usually observed as characteristic symptoms of the disease. (2) Slight narrowing of systemically infected leaves is also observed. (3) Pods also exhibit symptoms of mosaic and malformation. (4) Some strains under certain conditions cause systemic necrosis that spreads into various plant parts leading to black root syndrome and plant death.

Host Range

Natural hosts are *Phaseolus* species, *Lupinus luteus* and wild legumes like *Rhynchosia minima*. Experimental hosts are *Cicer aretinum, Glycine max, Trifolium incarnation* and *Vicia faba*. Non-leguminous hosts include *Nicotiana clevelandii* and *N. benthamiana*.

Transmission

The disease is seed borne in nature. Several aphid species including *Acyrthosiphon pisum, Aphis fabae* and *Myzus persicae* transmit the virus in non-persistent manner in the nature. Some other species of the aphids such as *Aphis gossypii, A. medicaginis* and *Macrosiphum pisi* have recently been reported to transmit the virus.

Management

(1) Only healthy seeds should be sown since seeds represent most important source of natural infection. (2) Plants for seed production should be grown in isolation from other susceptible legume crops and under conditions least favorable for aphid development. (3) Each infected plant should be rogued immediately from such crop upon detection. (4) Chemical control of the aphids for seed crop is also recommended.

5. Tomato Spotted Wilt Disease

The disease is caused by Tomato spotted wilt *tospovirus*.

The disease has been recorded from both temperate and sub-tropical regions of the world.

Symptoms

Initial symptoms are vein-swelling and appearance of necrotic ring spots on young leaves of the infected plants. The leaves twist upward or downward and become brittle. Stems also twist, shorten and in due course shoots are converted into bushy appearance. Suitable diagnostic plants are *Petunia hybrida* producing local necrotic spots without systemic infection and *Lycopersicon lycopersicum* in which inoculated leaves remain symptom-less and bronze patching are seen on leaves.

Host Range

Tomato, pepper, potato and egg plants are main hosts among vegetables. Other susceptible hosts include *Lactuca sativa*, *Phaseolus vulgaris*, *Pisum sativum*, *Vicia fabae*, *Nicotiana tabacum* and *Vigna sincenses*. Different species of flowers such as *Petunia*, *Begonia*, *Chrysanthemum*, *Dahilia* and *Zinnia* are also susceptible hosts.

Transmission

Thrips species are natural virus vectors. The insect acquires virus in their larval stage and transmits it only in the adult stage. The virus is not known to be transmitted trans-ovarially to the offspring.

Management

(1) Chemical control should be done to prevent excessive insect multiplication. (2) Tomato and pepper seedlings should be prepared in separate seed beds isolated from tobacco seedlings to avoid initial infection potential. (3) Besides these, other susceptible plants including weeds should be destroyed for successful management of this disease.

6. Tomato Yellow Leaf Curl Disease

The disease is caused by Tomato yellow leaf curl *begomovirus.*

The disease is more prevalent in Israel, Tunisia, Africa, India, Mexico, Venezuela and Europe.

Symptoms

Infected tomato plants are small, malformed, curled upward and severely chlorotic.

Host Range

Tomato (*Lycopersicon lycopersicum* and *L. esculentum*), *Datura strumonium* and *Malva* species are natural virus hosts.

Transmission

The whitefly, *Bemisia tabaci* transmits the virus in a circulative non-propagative manner.

Management

(1) Avoid continuous growing of tomato. (2) Practice crop rotation by planting crops that are not susceptible to whitefly. (3) Use resistant/tolerant varieties, *e.g.*

'Amareto', 'Peto 86', 'Fiona F1', 'Perlina', 'Denise', 'Cheyenne (E448)', 'Rover'. (4) Mulch the seedbeds. (5) Protect seedbeds with a white nylon net (40 mesh). (6) Pull out diseased seedlings. (7) Protect seedlings from whiteflies. (8) Plant barrier crops like maize around tomato fields. These crops should be sown a month or two before transplanting of tomato. (9) Mulch tomato fields with sawdust or straw. (10) Immediately remove infected plants and bury them. (11) Do not plant cotton near tomato and/or other crops susceptible to whiteflies or *vice versa*. (12) Eradicate weeds. (13) Plough-under all plant debris after harvest or burn them when possible.

7. Banana Bunchy Top Disease

The disease is caused by Banana bunchy top *nanavirus*.

The disease is known to occur in most of the banana growing regions throughout the world, including Australia, Asia, Pacific Islands and Africa. The virus causes complete destruction of plantations, if not controlled.

Symptoms

(1) Irregular dark green streaks develop along the leaf veins. (2) The leaves in the apical plant part are bunched as rosettes. (3) Infected plants grow slowly and fail to produce fruits.

Disease Cycle

The virus is preserved permanently in infected perennial banana and is transmitted naturally with infected suckers used as planting material. The

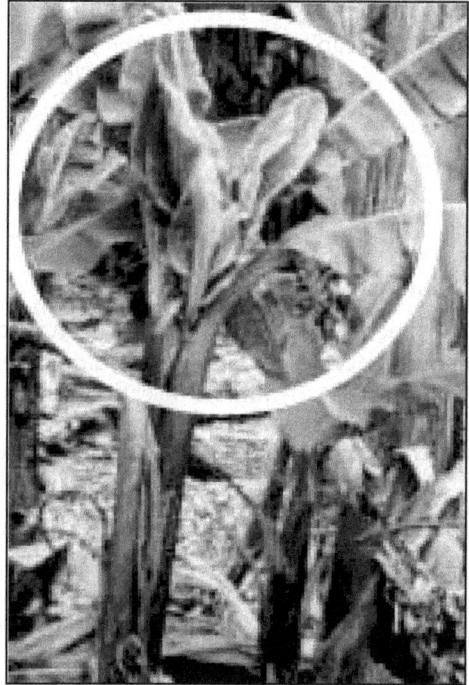

Figure 64: Banana Plants with Bunchy Top Symptoms.

banana aphid, *Pentalonia nigronevosa* transmits the virus in non-persistent manner.

Management

(1) Virus-free suckers should be used to establish new orchard. (2) Aphid vectors should be managed by using suitable insecticide. (3) Infected trees should be destroyed immediately upon detection. (4) Quarantine regulatory measures should be strictly followed to avoid introduction of virus infected planting materials into new areas.

8. Chilli Leaf Curl Disease

The disease is caused by Tobacco leaf curl *begomovirus*.

Leaf curl is the most destructive disease of chilli and it causes severe loss in yield every year in infected crop.

Symptoms

(1) The disease is characterized by the stunting of the plants with rolling and crinkling of leaves of the affected plants. (2) The newly formed leaves exhibit chlorosis and old curled leaves become leathery and brittle. (3) Dwarfing of the plants is usually due to shortening of the internodes. (4) Only few fruits are set and such fruits remain smaller and malformed.

Host Range

The virus has a wide host range. Transmission studies have showed that whiteflies can transmit the virus successfully to many hosts like *Nicotiana tabacum*, *N. glutinosa*, *Lycopersicum* species, *Petunia hybrida*, *Capsicum* species, and *Crotalaria juncea*.

Transmission

The virus is successfully transmitted by wedge grafting. The whitefly, *Bemisia tabaci* transmits the virus to *Capsicum* species and many other host plants.

Management

The crop must be protected from seedling to fruiting stage and diseased plants should be removed from the field on detection so as to avoid spread of the disease. Judicious use of suitable insecticide is also recommended.

Plant Diseases Caused by Viroids

Viroids are a unique class of plant pathogens. They solely consist of a small, single-stranded, circular RNA, which is not encapsidated in a protein coat. These naked RNA molecules cause serious diseases among many crop plants, fruit trees and ornamentals, including potato, tomato, cucumber, chrysanthemum, avocado, and coconut palms, to name only a few. The viroid-induced diseases lead to dramatic economic losses in agriculture and horticulture worldwide.

Viroids were discovered and given this name by Theodor Otto Diener, a plant pathologist at the Agricultural Research Service in Maryland, in 1971. The first viroid to be identified was the *potato spindle tuber viroid* (PSTVd).

1. Potato Spindle Tuber

This disease is caused by Potato Spindle Tuber Viroid (PSTVd).

Symptoms

(1) Growth of infected plants may be severely reduced or even cease entirely. (2) The vines of infected plants may be smaller, more upright, and produce smaller leaves than their healthy counterparts. (3) Infected tubers may be small, elongated, spindle-shaped (from which the disease derives its name), misshapen, and cracked. (4) Their eyes may be more pronounced than normal and may be borne on knob-like protuberances that may even develop into small tubers.

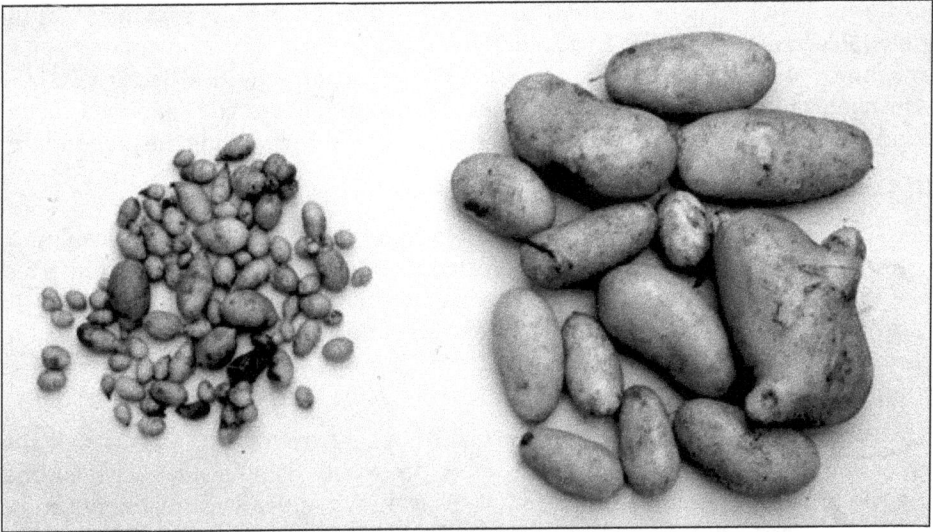

Figure 65: Tubers from Potato Plants Affected by Potato Spindle Tuber Viroid.

Host Range

The natural host range of PSTVd includes many solanaceous species. The viroid may cause disease in *Solanum tuberosum* (potato), *Lycopersicon esculentum* (tomato), and *Capsicum annuum* (pepper) where symptoms may vary considerably depending on plant species, variety, viroid strain and environmental conditions. Infections in other hosts are symptom-less; *e.g.*, *Brugmansia* spp., *Datura* sp., *S. rantonneti*, *Persea americana* (avocado), *Physalis peruviana* (cape gooseberry), *S. jasminoides*, *S. muricatum* (pepino), and *Streptosolen jamesonii*.

Transmission

PSTVd can be transmitted in four different ways *i.e.*, propagation by tubers, cuttings, and micro-plants provides a very efficient means of viroid transmission, under favorable conditions, PSTVd is readily transmitted by normal cultivation activities as clearly seen with potatoes and tomatoes, where viroid spread is mainly along the row, PSTVd is spread all over the world via infected true seed and transmission by aphids which requires the source plant to be infected by both Potato leaf roll virus (PLRV) and PSTVd.

Disease Management

Disease management can be divided into two parts:

A. *Prevention of Infection*

This includes all measures to prevent the introduction of PSTVd into a specific crop. It is very important to start a new cultivation with viroid-free planting material (tubers, seeds or plants). PSTVd is considered a quarantine 'organism' in many countries, and therefore, governmental measures to prevent introduction of PSTVd with plants from other countries will often be applied. Certification schemes including testing may be required to provide further guarantees that the planting material is free from PSTVd. In addition to the use of healthy planting material, it is also important to prevent viroid introduction via human activities. Because PSTVd is mechanically transmissible, it can be introduced into potential host plants via the hands, clothes, or equipment used by people working in or visiting the greenhouse.

B. Viroid Eradication

It is based on destruction of PSTVd-infected plants and thorough cleaning of equipment and greenhouses where infected plants have been grown. All infected plants together with those from an adequate buffer zone should be destroyed. In case of field-grown potatoes, crop rotations involving non-PSTVd host species help eliminate infected volunteer plants. In case of symptom-less infections such as those commonly observed in ornamentals, all plants in the lot should be destroyed.

When PSTVd is identified in a greenhouse-grown crop, all parts of the greenhouse should be thoroughly cleaned, preferably using a steam cleaner and a scrub brush for parts that are difficult to clean. A regular acid treatment can be used for watering tubes and drippers. After cleaning the greenhouse and associated equipment, application of a disinfectant completes the eradication procedure. When cultivation of crops susceptible to PSTVd infection resumes, extra monitoring for PSTVd symptoms and/or testing are advisable.

2. Chrysanthemum Stunt

This disease is caused by Chrysanthemum Stunt Viroid (CSVd), and is closely related to Potato Spindle Tuber Viroid (PSTVd) and Cucumber Pale Fruit Viroid.

Symptoms

In florists' chrysanthemums, about 30 per cent of plants are symptom-less carriers. However, even when symptoms are manifest, comparison with a healthy plant cannot always confirm diagnosis which, in general, can only be established by indexing on differential hosts. Infected plants bloom earlier than normal plants of the same cultivar and this effect increases with time; on plants coming from infected mother plants, it is usually shorter in the first year of infection (a few days) than in the following year (up to more than 3 weeks). Flowers are fewer and smaller and the colour, particularly of the bronze and red ones, may be bleached to a lighter shade.

Plants infected the previous summer produce far fewer laterals the following spring. Leaves are reduced in number and size; a striking crinkle symptom is found in cvs Blanche and Yellow Garza, the leaf surface being wavy or crumpled with associated yellowish-green patches. Stems become very brittle and break easily where they branch. CSVd is easily transmitted by mechanical means and also by *Cuscuta* sp.

Tanacetum parthenium cv. Matricaria Golden Ball may show a dwarfing with associated pale leaves and shortened, crowded inflorescences. *Chrysanthemum prealtum* may develop resetting.

Hosts

The main hosts of CSVd are florists' chrysanthemums (*Dendranthema morifolium*) and related ornamentals including *Chrysanthemum prealtum*, *D. indicum* and *Tanacetum parthenium*. Susceptibility varies between cultivars, but generally all-the-year-round cultivars are more susceptible.

Many other Asteraceae can be infected experimentally, such as: *Achillea* spp., *Ambrosia trifida*, *Anthemis tinctoria*, *Centaurea cyanus*, other *Chrysanthemum* spp., *Dahlia pinnata*, *Echinacea purpurea*, *Emilia javanica*, *Gynura aurantiaca*, *Heliopsis pitcheriana*, *Liatris pycnostachya*, *Senecio* spp., *Tanacetum* spp., *Venidium fastuosum* and *Zinnia elegans*. Of 39 species and cultivars found to be susceptible, only seven developed discernible symptoms.

Management

Control of the disease is extremely difficult due to its highly contagious nature and long latent period. Viroid-free plants may be obtained by meristem-tip culture, which may be combined with heat treatment. However, the proportion of viroid-free plants which can be obtained is only about 5 per cent. Planting material should be obtained from mother plants of third generation or less. Alternatively, the consignment should be derived from mother plants found free from CSVd at the time of flowering by inspection of 30 plants or 10 per cent of the consignment, whichever is the greater.

3. Citrus Exocortis

This disease is caused by Citrus Exocortis Viroid (CEVd). It can infect all varieties of citrus but is symptom-less in most.

Symptoms

Symptoms of exocortis develop on *P. trifoliate*, citrange and Swingle citrumelo rootstocks. Trees grown on *P. trifoliata* are the most severely affected, with symptoms of bark scaling and severe stunting usually developing when trees are around 4 years of age. When bark scaling occurs it appears as cracking and peeling of the bark below the bud union.

Trees grown on citrange rootstock develop symptoms slightly later and the degree of tree stunting is usually not as severe as that on *P. trifoliata*. Trees on citrange rootstocks do not always develop bark scaling. On other sensitive rootstocks, symptoms include tree stunting, yellowing of the canopy and general tree decline and occasional flaking of the bark of the rootstock. Exocortis has no effect on fruit quality but because it stunts trees it severely reduces tree yield. The type and severity of symptoms is dependent on the rootstock and the amount of exocortis viroid present in the scion, as well as the presence of other citrus viroids in the tree. High temperatures can also accelerate symptom development.

Disease Source and Spread

The viroid is carried in the plant sap and can be spread from tree to tree by budding or grafting activities and on pruning and hedging equipment. Natural grafting of tree roots can also transmit the viroid between trees. Exocortis is not transmitted by sap-sucking insects, as there is no known insect vector of the disease. Seed transmission is unknown. Ease of mechanical transmission also varies with the citrus scion, *e.g.* it is easier to transmit CEVd between lemons, than lemon to orange or orange to orange.

Management

Citrus trees showing symptoms of exocortis should be tested to verify the presence of the exocortis viroid. Any infected trees need to be removed from the orchard and destroyed so that the viroid is not transmitted to other trees or blocks. As much as possible the root system should be removed to prevent root sprouting. Trees infected with exocortis should not be used as a budwood source for the production of citrus trees. While purchasing citrus plants from a nursery, insist on disease-free certified grafts. Because CEVd can be mechanically transmitted on cutting, pruning or hedging equipment these implements need to be sterilised in a 1 per cent bleach solution (1 per cent available chlorine).

4. Coconut Cadang-Cadang

This disease is caused by Citrus Cadang-Cadang Viroid (CCCVd).

Hosts

Coconuts, *Corypha elata* and oil palms (*Elaeis guineensis*). In addition, arecanuts, *Chrysalidocarpus lutescens*, dates, *Ptychosperma macarthurii*, *Roystonea regia* and *Veitchia merrillii* are susceptible to inoculation with CCCVd. CCCVd-like sequences have also been identified in some symptomless herbaceous monocotyledonous species growing near CCCVd-infected coconuts.

Symptoms: *Early stage (lasting 2-4 years)*: Yellow leaf spots appearing water-soaked in reflected light, translucent yellow in transmitted light. Nuts become small and rounded, with characteristic equatorial scarifications. *Medium stage (lasting around 2 years)*: Leaf spots become numerous, giving the lower two-thirds of the crown a yellowish appearance. Inflorescences become necrotic, infertile and nut production ceases. Frond production and size decline. *Late stage (lasting around 5 years)*: Leaf spots almost confluent. Whole crown yellow/bronze-coloured and much reduced in size and number of fronds. Leaflets become brittle and palm dies. Time from appearance of first symptoms to tree death ranges from around 8 to 16 years and is generally greater in older palms.

Disease Source and Spread

The viroid has been detected in the husk and embryo of nuts and can be seed transmitted, but only at a low frequency. Mechanical transmission through wounds caused by cultural practices or insect feeding wounds might also occur.

Management

No known control measures exist for CCCVd in the field. Specific control recommendations cannot be developed until the epidemiology of CCCVd is more clearly understood. Potential control strategies include elimination of reservoir species, vector control, mild strain protection and breeding for host resistance. Eradication of diseased plants is usually performed to minimize spread but is of dubious efficacy due to the difficulties of early diagnosis.

Phytosanitary Measures

CCCVd certainly has potential pest significance on many species of palms, grown as outdoor or indoor ornamentals. Ideally, no imported palm seed or propagating material (including embryo cultures) should be moved into diseases-free region from infested countries unless it is shown to be free from viroids by molecular diagnostic methods.

8

Plant Diseases Caused by Fastidious Vascular Bacteria (Rickettssia like Organisms)

Fastidious vascular bacteria are similar to bacteria in all respects but are obligate parasites (or) unable to grow on conventional bacteriological media.

☆ Rickettssia were discovered by 'Howard Taylor Ricket'.

☆ First time observed in 1972 in phloem of cloves and periwrinkle plants affected with clover club leaf disease.

Important Characteristics

☆ Thin cell walls with 20-30 nm thickness.

☆ Generally rods and pleomorphic.

☆ Size 1-4 nm long and 0.2-0.8 nm diameter.

☆ No flagella, hence non-motile.

☆ All are gram-negative except, sugarcane ratoon stunt which is gram-positive.

☆ Non-spore formers.

☆ Reproduce by Binary fission.

☆ Occur in xylem and phloem vessels.

☆ Intracellular obligate parasites except xylem habitant gram-positive sugarcane ratoton stunt RLO.

☆ Transmission only by mechanical means.

☆ Vectors for phloem inhabitants are psyilids.

☆ Sensitive to high temperature, hence can be eliminated by treating the propagating material with hot water at 45°-50°C for 4-8 hours.

Important Diseases and Transmission

1) Wilt in Potato, Tomato and Alfalfa – *Clavibacter* sps.

☆ Xylem inhabitant, gram-positive.

☆ Transmission - no vector, only sap transmission.

☆ Can be grown on complex nutrient medium.

2) Citrus Greening – *Liberobacter asiaticus*

☆ Phloem inhabitant, gram-negative.

☆ Rigid rods, obligate parasites.

☆ Transmission – *Diaphorinia citri* (Psyllids) and vegetative propagation.

9

Plant Diseases Caused by Mollicutes

Doi *et al.*, (Japan) in 1967, observed some wall-less micro-organisms in the phloem of rice plant infected with yellows type disease and named them as **P**leuro **P**neumonia-Like **O**rganisms (PPLO) or **M**ycoplasma Like **O**rganisms (MLOs). Ishie *et al.*, (Japan) in the same year reported that mulberry dwarf disease also caused by MLOs can be controlled by with tetracycline antibiotics.

Recently, the MLOs infecting plants were designated as *Phytoplasmas*. Phytoplasmas are obligate, pleomorphic non-helical, wall-less but surrounded by a triple layered unit membrane, phloem-limited, prokaryotic, non-helical mollicutes that can infect plants and cannot be grown in culture medium.

Phytoplasmas with helical shape that can be cultured on cell-free medium are called **spiroplasmas**.

Phytoplasmas are included in the Kingdom Bacteria and classified under the Phylum Firmicutes or Tenericutes and **Class Mollicutes** as they resemble the L-form bacteria without cell walls and other mollicutes infecting various animals including man. The best-known genus in mollicutes is *Mycoplasma.* The word "Mollicutes" is derived from the Latin word *mollis* (meaning "soft" or "pliable"), and *cutis* (meaning "skin").

Important Characteristics of Phytoplasmas

☆ Unicellular, obligate, prokaryotic micro-organisms inhabiting phloem sieve tubes of plants.

☆ Lack cell wall but bound by trilamellar unit membrane made of lipo-protein.

☆ Pleomorphic.

☆ Osmotically stable.

☆ Self-replicable, multiply by binary fission.

☆ Non-flagellate, non-spore former, gram-negative.

☆ Sensitive to tetracycline, chloromphenical but resistant to penicillin.

☆ Transmitted mainly by leaf happens and also by grafting and dodder.

☆ Filterable through bacteria-proof filters.

☆ Infected by virus.

☆ Requires sterols for growth.

☆ No family and genera have been designated so far.

Important Plant Diseases Caused by Phytoplasmas and their Vectors

Diseases	Vector
Aster yellows	*Macrosteles fascifrons* and *M. quadrilineatus*
Little leaf of Brinjal	*Hishimonus phycitis*
Potato witches' broom	*Scleroracus flavopictus*

Spiroplasmas

Spiroplasmas are helical, wall-less prokaryotic micro-organisms that are present in phloem of diseased plants, often helical in culture and are thought to be kind of mycoplasmas, but can be cultured on artificial medium. Bove *et al.,* (1968) first time identified spiroplasmas as causal agent of corn smut.

Important Characteristics of Spiroplasmas

☆ Helical in shape.

☆ Can be grown on culture medium.

☆ Gram-positive.

☆ Growth on culture medium appears as fried eggs colonies.

Important Plant Diseases Caused by Spiroplasmas and their Vectors

Diseases	Vector
Citrus stubborn (*Spiroplasma citri*)	*Circulifer tenellus*
Corn smut (*Spiroplasma kunkeli*)	*Dalbulus maidis*

10

Plant Diseases Caused by Protozoa and Algae

Certain trypanosomatid flagellates belonging to the Kingdom Protozoa, Phylum Euglenozoa, Order Kinetoplastidae, and Family Trypanosomatidae, have been known to parasitize plants since the early 1900s. That flagellates may be pathogenic to their host plants was suggested several times by the investigators of these parasites, and rather good evidence was presented that some plant diseases are caused by flagellates. As these parasites could not be isolated in pure culture and could not be inoculated into healthy plants so that they could reproduce the disease, as Koch's rules dictate, flagellates have not yet been fully accepted as plant pathogens. Nevertheless, the pathogenicity of phytoplasmas and of some fastidious vascular bacteria in plants is almost universally accepted, although the same Koch's rules are equally unfulfilled with these organisms as with the flagellates.

The protozoa are mostly one-celled, microscopic organisms, generally motile, and have typical nuclei. They may live alone or in colonies and may be free-living, symbiotic, or parasitic.

Flagellates are characterized by one or more long slender flagella at some or all stages of their life cycle. Although many flagellates are saprophytic and some contain plastids with colored pigments, including functional chlorophyll, others are parasites with some causing serious diseases of humans and various animals.

Nomenclature of Plant Trypanosomatids

Flagellate protozoa were first found to be associated with plants in 1909, in Mauritius, when Lafont reported that the protozoa parasitize the latex-bearing cells (the laticifers) of the laticiferous plant *Euphorbia* (Euphorbiaceae). To distinguish them from protozoa parasitizing humans and animals, plant protozoa were placed in a new genus, *Phytomonas*, and the one described by Lafont was named *P. davidi.* Since then several other species of *Phytomonas* have been reported from plants belonging to the families Asclepiadaceae (*e.g., P. elmassiani* on milkweed); Moraceae (*e.g., P. bancrofti* on *Ficus* spp.); Rubiaceae (*e.g., P. leptovasorum* on coffee); and Euphorbiaceae (*e.g., P. francai* on cassava). Unnamed species have been reported on coconut and oil palm; and on the ornamental plant, red ginger *Alpinia purpurata* of the Zingiberaceae. All plant flagellates belong to the Order Kinetoplastida, Family Trypanosomatidae. In recent years, however, flagellate protozoa have been isolated from fruits such as tomato. These flagellates, although trypanosomatids, do not seem to all belong to the genus *Phytomonas*.

Taxonomy of Plant Trypanosomatids

The taxonomy of *Phytomonas* species has not yet been resolved. The genus *Phytomonas* includes promastigote, trypanosomatid flagellate members that are parasites and have a life cycle completed in two hosts, a plant and an insect. In plants, some *Phytomonas* species live in the phloem sieve tubes of non-laticiferous plants, such as coconut and oil palms, red ginger and coffee, and are definitely pathogenic. Others live in the latex-containing cells of laticiferous plants and are not considered to be pathogenic, although one (*P. francai*) has been associated with the empty root and subsequent decline of cassava. Still other trypanosomatid flagellates, some are *Phytomonas* species while others do not belong to *Phytomonas* but parasitize and cause damage only to the fruits and seeds of several plants.

Plant Diseases Caused by Phloem-Restricted Trypanosomatids

These include the main plant diseases caused by trypanosomatids. They have several common characteristics. Coffee phloem necrosis was apparently quite widespread in northern South America but its present distribution is uncertain. The palm diseases, hart-rot of coconut palm and marcitez sopresiva of oil palm, occur wherever these plants are grown north of Lima, Peru, up to Brazil, Trinidad, and Honduras. Red ginger wilt and decay have been found only in the Caribbean island of Grenada.

1. Phloem Necrosis of Coffee

Phloem necrosis of coffee occurs in Surinam, Guyana and probably Brazil, San Salvador and Colombia. It affects *Coffea liberica, C. arabica* and other species. Infected trees show sparse foliage, yellowing, and dropping of leaves. As the symptoms advance gradually, only the young top leaves remain on the otherwise bare branches. The roots begin to die back and the condition of the tree worsens with eventual death of the tree. Sometimes at the beginning of the dry season, trees wilt and die within 3 or 6 weeks. The roots and trunk of trees show multiple divisions of cambial cells internally, and production of a zone of smaller and shorter phloem vessels of disorderly structure right next to the wood cylinder. At this stage the bark in the roots and the trunk is firmly attached to the wood and cannot be separated from it.

The flagellates can be traced from the roots upward into the trunk, where they seem to migrate vertically in the phloem and laterally through the sieve plates into healthy sieve tubes. They also seem to move downward into unaffected roots. The disease can be transmitted through root grafts but not through green branch or leaf grafts.

2. Hart-Rot and Sudden Wilt of Coconut Palms

Hart-rot has been known in Surinam since 1906 under the more appropriate names *viz.*, lethal yellowing or bronze-leaf wilt. The disease also occurs in Colombia and Ecuador and under the local name Cedros wilt in Trinidad.

The symptoms of hart-rot include yellowing and browning of the tips of older leaves that subsequently spread to younger leaves. Recently opened inflorescences are black whereas unripe nuts of symptomatic trees drop. At this stage, root tips also begin to rot. Petioles of older leaves may break, and the spear becomes necrotic. At later stages, the apical region of the crown also rots and often produces a foul odor. Trees infected with hart-rot die within one to a few months of the appearance of external symptoms.

Hart-rot causing protozoa are transmitted by pentatomid insects of the genera *Lincus* and *Ocblerus*. Hart-rot spreads very rapidly. For example, about 15,000 coconut trees died in three years in the Cedros region of Trinidad.

3. Sudden Wilt (*Marchitez sopresiva*) of Oil Palm

Sudden wilt of oil palms is rather common and widespread in northern South America. It has been known since the 1960s in Colombia. The disease spreads rapidly through oil palm plantations and causes considerable damage by killing trees first in loci of a few to many trees and then in increasingly larger areas.

Symptoms begin as browning of the tips of the lower leaf leaflets. The browning subsequently spreads to the upper leaves and eventually becomes ash gray. In the meantime, root tips also begin to die, and the whole root system deteriorates. As a result, plant growth slows down, fruit bunches discolor and rot or fall off. Within a few weeks all leaves become ash gray and dry up and the whole tree dies. *Phytomonas* flagellates occur widely in the phloem sieve elements of roots, leaves, and inflorescences of infected plants. These flagellates are also transmitted readily by the pentatomid insects *Lincus* and *Ochlerus*.

Some control of sudden wilt has reportedly been obtained by spraying insecticides that control the vectors of the protozoa.

Plant Diseases Caused by Laticifer-Restricted Trypanosomatids

Empty Root of Cassava (*Manihot esculenta*)

Trypanosomatids growing in the latex of laticiferous plants have been found almost worldwide in plants belonging to at least nine families. Latex trypanosomatids are transmitted from plant to plant by pentatomid bugs from the genera *Lincus*, *Ochlerus*, and probably others.

Infected laticiferous plants generally show no pathological symptoms, but in the case of empty root of cassava, a laticiferous plant, symptoms are produced. The empty root disease was observed affecting certain cultivars of cassava in the Espirito Santo state of Brazil. The root system of affected plants develops poorly. Roots in general remain small and slender and contain little or no starch. The above ground parts of infected plants show general chlorosis and decline. The empty root disease can be transmitted by grafting. It also spreads rapidly in the field, probably by pentatomid insects.

Plant Diseases Caused by Fruit- and Seed-Infecting Trypanosomatids

Fruit Trypanosomatids

Trypanosomatids have been found to cause minor disease on tomatoes in South Africa, Spain and Brazil. At least four genera of trypanosomatids have been isolated from tomato fruit but so far all are called *Phytomonas serpens*.

The disease appears as localized yellow patches that may also exhibit malformations and it is within these patches that trypanosomatids can be found multiplying in the wound made by the insect vector.

General Characters and Classification of Phytopathogenic Algae

Algae are unicellular or multicellular, eukaryotic (except Cyanophyceae), chlorophyllous, autotrophic, thalloid organisms. The study of algae is called "**Phycology**". So far 18,000 genera and 29,000 species have been identified. These are pioneer plants and main oxygen evolvers. They show large diversity in every aspect.

Generally, algae were classified on the basis of photosynthetic pigments, nature of storage of food material, nature of cell wall components, cell structure and types of flagella. Though many classifications were made by different scientists still Fritch classification is a widely accepted one. According to this classification, algae have been classified into 11 classes. Algae exhibit wide diversity in the thallus organization. They range in unicellular, non-motile to multi-cellular, motile forms. Algae carry reproduction by means of vegetative, asexual and sexual methods. They also show variability in their life cycles. The most primitive life cycle is haplontic and the most advance life cycle is diplobiontic.

Scientific Classification of *Cephaleuros virescens*

Kingdom: Plantae
Phylum: Chlorophyta
Class: Incertae sedis
Subclass: Incertae sedis
Order: Trentepohliales
Family: Trentepohliacease
Genus: *Cephaleuros*
Species: *C. virescens*

Algal Leaf Spot (Red Rust)

Algal leaf spot, caused by the alga *Cephaleuros virescens*, may appear on a wide variety of plant species. The list of plants susceptible to *C. virescens* includes apple, mango, jasmine, juniper, oak, guava, sapota etc.

Symptoms

Leaf spots develop as pale green or pale red, rough, superficial, netlike circular spots with wavy or feathered margins. In some situations and on some hosts, the alga may infect twigs and branches, causing girdling lesions. Algal infections of twigs often cause superficial cell layers to become slightly swollen and cracked; this cracking will cause the twigs to be more susceptible to fungal infection. When sporangia (algal spore structures) are produced, the lesions become reddish. When sporangia are not produced, the spots remain light green in color.

Persistence and Transmission

Disease spread is favored by frequent rains. During wet weather, spores are spread by water droplets or wind-driven rain to leaves or twigs which are then colonized by the alga. *Cephaleuros virescens* can survive adverse conditions in spots on leaves and twigs. Weakened trees or plants are most susceptible to attack by the alga.

Management

Copper oxychloride @ 0.3 per cent was found most effective in reducing the disease. The fungicides, captafol (0.2 per cent) and ziram (0.25 per cent) are also effective.

11

Phanerogamic Parasites

Although most of the plant diseases are caused by fungi, bacteria, viruses and others, there are a few seed plants (phanerogams) which are parasitic on living plants. More than 2500 species of higher plants are known to live parasitically on other plants. These parasitic plants produce flowers and seeds similar to those produced by the plants they parasitize. Some of these parasites attack roots of the host while others parasitize the stem. Some are devoid of chlorophyll and depend entirely upon their host for food supply while others have chlorophyll and obtain only the minerals and water from the host for photosynthesis.

The parasitic flowering plants may be grouped as follows:

1. Stem parasites:
    a. Complete parasite – Dodders – *Cuscuta* and *Cassytha*
    b. Partial parasite – Mistletoes – *Loranthus* and *Dendrophthoe*
2. Root parasites:
    a. Complete parasite – Broom rape - *Orabanche*
    b. Partial parasite – Witch weed - *Striga*

A. Dodder – *Cuscuta* sp.

Cuscuta and *cassytha* are slender, twining plants. The stem is tough, curling, thread-like and leafless, bearing only minute scales in place of leaves. The stem is usually yellowish or orange in color, sometimes tinged with red or purple; sometimes it is almost white. Tiny flowers massed in clusters occur on the stem. Grey to reddish brown seeds is produced in abundance by the flowers and mature within a few weeks from bloom. The seeds fall to the ground and may germinate immediately or may remain dormant and germinate in the following growth reason when conditions are favourable. Mango, citrus, clover, berseem, flax and many other crops are commonly parasitized.

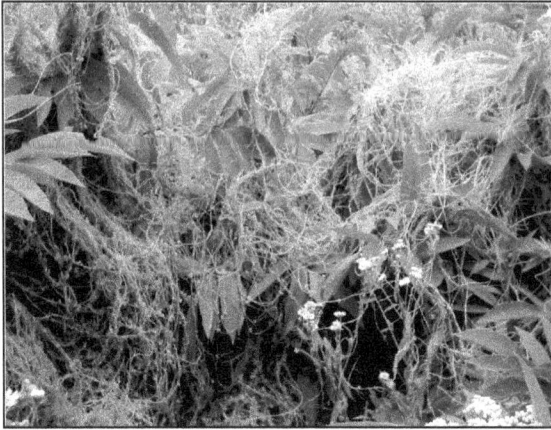

Figure 66: *Cuscuta* sp.

B. Mistletoes – *Loranthus* sp.; *Dendrophthoe* sp.

These plants are strongly branched and glabrous shrubs. The stem is thick, erect, flattened at the nodes and appears to arise in clusters at the point of attachment to the host. The place at which the host is attacked and where the haustorium penetrates often swells to form tumors which vary in size according to age of the parasite. The flowers are borne in clusters. They are long and tubular in shape and usually greenish white or red in color. The fruit is fleshy and contains a solitary seed. It is sweet and eaten by birds and animals. The parasite is spread by dispersal of its seed mostly through birds and to some extent by other animals. Conifers, Mango, Citrus and other fruit trees are commonly attacked.

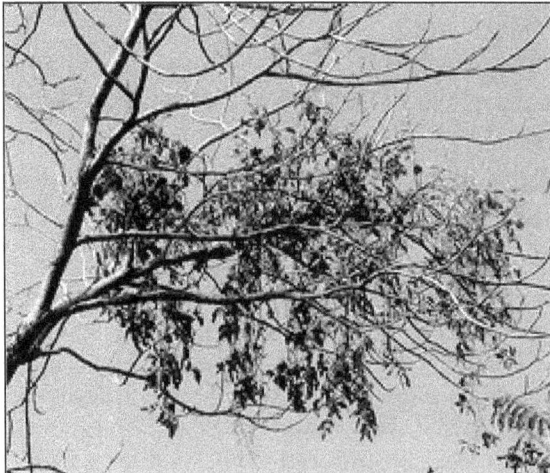

Figure 67: *Loranthus* sp.

C. Broom Rape – *Orabanche cernua*

The parasite consists of a stout, fleshy stem, 10-15 inches long. The stem is pale yellow to brownish red in color and is covered by small, thin and brown scaly leaves. Flowers appearing in the axils of leaves are white and tubular. The seeds are very small and black and may remain viable in the soil for several years. It affects tobacco, brinjal, tomato, cabbage, cauliflower and turnip and many other crops.

D. Witch Weed – *Striga lutea*

It is a small plant with bright green stem and leaves. Both stem and leaves are slightly hairy. The weed grows 15-30 cm high and produces multiple branches both near the ground and

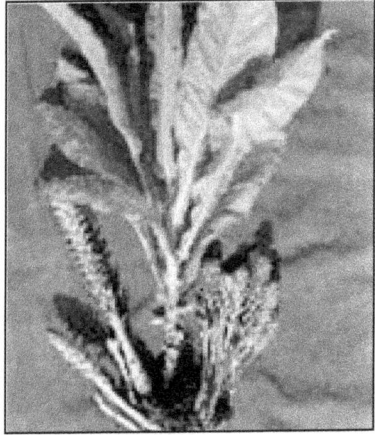

Figure 68: *Orabanche cernua* on Tobacco.

higher on the plant. The leaves are long and narrow and grow opposite to each other in pairs; each pair being at 90° to the preceding one. The flowers are small and usually brick red. A single plant may produce from 50,000 to 500,000 seeds. It attacks sugarcane, rice, sorghum, maize and some grasses.

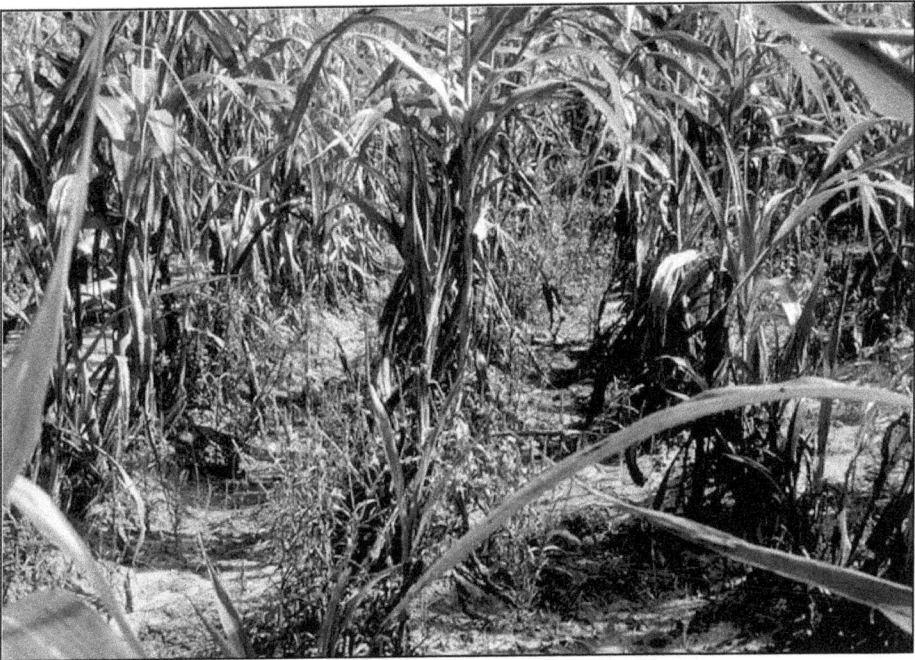

Figure 69: *Striga hermonthica* spp. on Maize.

12

Non-Parasitic Diseases

The abiotic factors sometimes cause injury to plant which is different from disease. Problems like mineral excesses or deficiencies, herbicide damage, salinity, light and temperature effects. Climatic effects and effects of soil physics and chemistry are some of the abiotic factors that cause injury to the plants.

Air Pollution

Stack gases emitted from the industrial processes and automobile exhausts are toxic to plants. Ozone and **peroxyacetyl** nitrate (PAN) are the most important. The symptom due to ozone damage is bleaching of area on the upper leaf surface. Ex. "Weather fleck" on tobacco.

Toxic Effects of Improperly Used Chemicals

Incorrect use of fertilizer, fungicide, weedicide and pesticide can cause serious damage. *e.g.* 2,4-D damage in cotton.

Black Tip of Mango

It is due to toxic gases produced from brick kilns nearer to the orchards. At the tip of the fruits, etiolation occurs and then it turns brown, enlarges and becomes black. Then the skin cracks exposing the flesh. The toxic gases disturb boron metabolism.

Temperature

Sudden rise or fall in temperature causes injury. Harmful effects of chilling, freezing and sunburn are well-known examples.

a. Chilling injury causes surface pitting, necrosis and failure in ripening of fruits.

b. Freezing injury is caused by formation of ice. Since water is more pure in intercellular spaces, ice crystals are first formed, the crystals damage various cell organelles.

c. Sun-scald: This occurs when shade loving plants are suddenly exposed to direct sun. Sunken brown areas on appled, water-soaked areas on tomatoes are examples of high temperature.

Heart Rot of Potato

It is due to poor aeration in storage. The central core of the potato tuber turns black and becomes hard. Such tubers will not be germinated in the field.

Important Non-pathogenic Diseases and their Management

1. Blossom End Rot of Tomato

The disease of tomato fruit is a nutritional disorder caused by a derangement of the water balance between the leaves and the fruits during the development of the plant. It is characterized by a lesion at the blossom end of the fruit, which occurs while the latter is still green or while it is ripening on the vine. A water-soaked spot appears at the point of attachment of the senescent petals. It enlarges quite rapidly until it is about 2 cm or more in diameter, and at the same time, the diseased tissue shrinks, depressing the surface of the lesion. The color of the fruit becomes darker and secondary organisms generally invade the tissues. The diseased portion of the fruit becomes delimited as a sunken, leathery, dark colored area.

Management

The most obvious method of controlling blossom end rot is to maintain an equable environment and to keep the soil uniformly moist. This should be taken care of, especially when the fruit begins to develop.

2. Black Heart of Potato

The centers of potato tubers with black heart show black portions when sliced open, or after being sliced open the potato tubers undergo a fairly rapid change in color from white or pink to brown or dark brown or black. Bartholomew (1915) has studied the progress of the disease. When a tuber exposed to 40°C for 24 hours is cut open, the interior tissue appears normal in the beginning, but upon exposure to air, pink discoloration occurs which gradually becomes dark brown or black. This was shown to be an enzymatic effect in which some of the amino acids, particularly tyrosine, pass through a series of intermediate compounds to the deeply colored, relatively stable and insoluble compounds known as melanin.

High temperatures bring about sub-oxidation by stimulating respiration under conditions in which cells in the interior of the tubers cannot secure an adequate supply of oxygen. Poorly ventilated storage over long periods predisposes potatoes to black heart.

Management

The disease can be significantly controlled by avoiding very high or low temperatures and by properly storing potatoes in well ventilated storage structures.

3. Mango Necrosis or Black Tip

Black tip of mango is characterized by the necrosis of one-third or half of the fruit. The most susceptible varieties are 'Dasheri', 'Safeda' and 'Langra'. The disease starts as a small, circular, pale patch at the tip of the mango fruit and soon enlarges, becomes black and covers the tip of the mango completely. The outer skin of the affected portion becomes flat and hard. Internally, in the vessels of the mesocarp, certain brown deposits are found which have been provisionally identified as tannins, flavotannins, flavophenols or their derivatives.

Previously it was thought that black kiln fumes are direct cause of the disease. Sen (1943), Das Gupta and Verma (1939), Das Gupta and Sinha (1944), working on the disease in Bihar and Uttar Pradesh, suggested that the smoke of black kiln fumes pollute the air with toxic gases such as sulphur dioxide and that these fumes caused the necrosis of the fruit tissues.

Management

The disease can be controlled by spraying borax at 2.7 kg/100 gallons three times in the season, *viz.*, pre-flowering, and flowering and immediately after fruit setting.

4. Zinc Deficiency Disease of Citrus

This disease is very common in many citrus gardens in India. It is also known as mottling or foliocellosis.

Symptoms

The main symptom is the production of alternate chlorotic regions and dark green patches in the leaf. The portions near the leaf veins are usually brown and the rest of the leaf is chlorotic. As a result of continual deficiency of zinc in the soil, there is severe stunting of the plant, reduction in leaf size, narrowing of the leaf lamina and severe chlorosis. The fruit size is also reduced. The plants become weak and are exposed to root infections and this slowly results in their death.

Management

As the application of zinc sulphate to the soil gives a very slow response, spraying zinc sulphate and lime mixture (zinc sulphate 2.268 kg and quick lime 2.268 kg in 100 gallons of water) is recommended for a quick response.

13

Pathogenesis

Pathogenesis is the sequence of processes in disease development that describes a pathogen's association with its host. The sequence begins with initial contact between the pathogen and host and ends when the pathogen is no longer associated with that host (*i.e.*, when the host/pathogen dies or the pathogen moves to another host). It can conveniently be divided into two parts *viz.*, infection process; and development of symptoms and signs. Symptoms are the expression of the host as a reaction to the infection and signs are the structures of the pathogen that are evident on the diseased areas of the host.

The Process of Infection

Infection is a process in which a pathogen enters, invades or penetrates a host plant and establishes parasitic relationship with it. The process starts with the inoculum reaching the host. The inoculum of most pathogens is carried over to the host plants either actively (or) passively to initiate the process of infection. Besides availability of a susceptible host and favorable environmental factors, viable inoculum is the most important factor for successful infection by the pathogen. During infection, pathogen grows, multiplies and colonizes the plant.

Inoculum: The pathogen (or) its parts that cause infection to the host.

Host: A plant that is infected by a parasite and from which the parasite obtains its nourishment.

Primary infection: The initial infection of the crop plants occurring for the first time in the crop season from the source of survival of the pathogen.

Primary inoculum: The propagules that cause primary infection are called primary inoculum. Normally these propagules are result of disease during previous season and survive to initiate fresh disease in the succeeding new season.

Secondary infection: After initiation of disease during the crop season through primary infection, the resultant spores/other propagating material produced by the pathogen are disseminated by different agencies and cause infection during the same crop season is called secondary infection.

Secondary inoculum: The propagules produced out of primary infection that cause secondary infection are called secondary inoculum. The rate of production of secondary inoculum by repeated cycles and the existence of favorable weather conditions decide the occurrence of epidemics.

The whole process of infection can be divided into 3 phases:

1. Pre-penetration phase;
2. Penetration phase; and
3. Post-penetration phase.

1) Pre-penetration Phase

This phase includes all events prior to actual entry of pathogen into the host. Before penetration, the pathogen must reach the host surface. The area of the host surface on which the inoculum lands or reaches for infection is called *'infection court'* and the process is called *'inoculation'*.

Fungi: The process starts with contact of spores with host surface. The fungal spores on germination, put out a small tube like structure called *'germ tube'*, which grows and attaches to the host surface with the help of a specialized structure *'appressorium'*.

The appressoria are formed when the germ tube touches the hard surface of the host due to *'hygrotropic'* response.

Ex: *Armillarialla mellea*.

Nematodes: Nematodes do not have any pre-penetration activities since they cannot multiply outside living host. The eggs of nematode hatch giving rise to second stage juveniles, which penetrate the host plant. The stylets are used to pierce the cell wall and the nematode body can enter the cell.

Bacteria: Bacteria also do not have any pre-penetration activities since they enter through wounds (or) natural openings. They multiply in the water drop on natural opening or sap on wounds.

Ex: *Xanthomonas campestris* pv. *campestris* causes 'black rot of crucifers' by entering through '**hydathodes**'.

Fastidious vascular bacteria, mollicutes, viruses, viroids, phytoplasmas etc.: Also do not have any penetration activities since they enter the host passively. They are placed directly into the cells of plants by their vectors (or) enter through wounds.

2) Penetration Phase

This is the actual entry of pathogen into their host plants. After coming in contact with the host, the pathogen proceeds to penetrate the host by breaking down structural (or) chemical barriers and establish physiological relationship with the host.

Pathogen penetrates the host in two different ways *viz.,* i) Indirect penetration and ii) Direct penetration.

i) Indirect Penetration

a) *Artificial openings like wounds*: The pathogens that enter the plants through wounds are called wound parasites. Wounds are caused by physical means such as implements used in various operations. All bacteria, most fungi, some viruses, fastidious vascular bacteria and all viroids can enter the plants through various types of wounds. In nature, viruses, viroids and mollicutes enter the plant through wound made by their vectors.

Ex: *Rhizopus, Aspergillus, Agrobacterium*

b) *Natural openings*: Many fungi and bacteria and some nematodes enter the plants through natural operations like stomata, lenticels and hydathodes. These openings are not covered by cuticle and thus important in providing direct access to the underlying tissues.

Fungal spores germinate on plant surface and the germ tube at its end develops an appressorium over the stomatal opening. A wedge-like structure grows from the appressorium into the stomatal opening and either forms a sub-stomatal vesicle or may directly penetrate through haustoria. Bacteria present in a film of water enter into leaves through stomata into sub-stomatal cavity or through hydathodes; into blossoms through nectar; and into fruits and stem through lenticels.

e.g. 1. Stomata:

Peronospora destructor - causing onion downy mildew;

Erwinia amylovora – causing fire blight of apple;

Meloidogyne incognita – root knot nematode of vegetables.

2. Lenticles: *Streptomyces scabies* – causing common scab of potato.

3. Hydathodes: *Xanthomonas campestris* pv. *campestris* – causing black rot of crucifers.

ii) Direct Penetration

The process of direct penetration is more complicated than entry through natural opening. The pathogen enters the host on its own efforts either mechanically (or) chemically breaking the host barriers like biochemical substances containing antimicrobial compounds. However, nature has provided the plants with different mechanisms of defense against attack by pathogens and their entry into the plant system. Direct penetration into intact plant surfaces like cuticle, epidermis, root hairs, flowers, etc., is the most common type of penetration in fungi and nematodes.

Besides mechanical force through appressorium and infection pegs, the fungi also produce various harmful substances like toxins, enzymes to overcome the chemical barriers produced by host, while the nematodes penetrate using mechanical force through their stylets.

The viruses cause infection only by direct contact with host protoplasm. They have no physical force (or) enzyme system of their own to overcome structural and/or chemical barriers of the host and come in contact with host only through wounds (or) insect vectors.

e.g.: Root hairs: *Fusarium oxysporum* f.sp. *conglutinanas* causing cabbage yellows.

Flower: *Claviceps microcephala* causing ergot of cereals;

Nectaries: *Erwinia amylovora* causing fire blight of apples;

Epidermal cells: *Venturia inequalis* causing apple scab.

3) Post-penetration Phase

This is the development of pathogen *i.e.*, colonization in plant after penetration and constitutes the last stage in pathogenesis in which the pathogen establishes the parasitic relationship with the host. The pathogen grows and multiplies within plant tissue and colonizes the plant resulting in disintegration or deterioration of invaded tissue producing symptoms. Different pathogens take varying periods of time in establishing within the host. Thus the incubation period vary from a few days to weeks under different environmental conditions. The colonization by plant pathogens in the host is several kinds.

1. **Ecto-parasites:** Mycelium lies superficially on surface of infected part with haustoria entering the epidermal cells. Ex: Powdery mildews, sooty molds etc.

2. **Endo-parasites wih external mycelium:** Some fungi are present inside the host and also produce external mycelium. Ex: *Corticium solani, Gauemannomyces graminis, Fomes annosus.*

3. **Sub-cuticular development:** The hyphae grow mostly between the cuticle and outer wall of epidermal cell. Ex: *Venturia inaequalis, Diplocarpon rosae.*

4. **Parenchymatous tissues:** Many pathogens colonize the parenchyma of cortex and mesophyll. Ex: *Taphrina* spp., *Pythium debaryanum, Phytophthora* spp., *Peronosporaceae, Albuginaceae,* rusts etc.

5. **Vascular tissues:** Vascular tissues are colonized by Hymenomycetes, some ascomycetes, deuteromycetes and bacteria. Both parenchyma and vessels of xylem are colonized. They cause wilt and rot diseases.

6. **Endobiotic development:** Fungi as *Olpidium, Plasmodiophora,* viruses, some bacteria grow exclusively inside the host cells.

7. **Systemic development:** They are highly specialized parasites. They have haustoria for nutrients and cause slight damage to tissue until later in life cycle. Some rusts, downy mildews, white rusts and smuts are good examples.

14

Survival and Dispersal of Plant Pathogens

In the absence of the host the pathogens survive to successfully continue the infection chain or diseases cycle. The pathogens have evolved a great variety of survival mechanisms during the period when the host is not available in the field.

The following terms are useful to understand the survival of plant pathogens.

Infection chain: Guamann (1950) has used the term *infection chain* for chain of events leading to the completion of pathogenesis over continuous crop seasons or Disease cycle.

The infection chain may be continuous or discontinuous (intermittent).

i) *Continuous infection chain*: The pathogen continuously survives in an active form by dispersal from one host plant to another host causing infection. Diseases caused by viruses and some of fungal and bacterial diseases have this type of infection chain.

ii) *Intermittent infection chain*: After harvest of crop the pathogen survives as dormant resting structures like spores, sclerotia and chlamydospores or as saprophytes to maintain continuity of infection chain. This is found in diseases caused by fungi, bacterium and nematodes.

The infection chain has 3 components *viz.*, survival, dissemination and infection.

Survival

The pathogens survive to sustain the infection chain in different ways. The sources of survival of plant pathogens can be grouped as:

A) Infected host (including plant or vector) as a source of inoculum.

B) Saprophytic survival outside the host.

C) Dormant spores/structures in or on the host or outside the host.

A) Infected Host Serving as a Reservoir of Active Inoculum

The host, on which the pathogen is over-summering (surviving during unfavorable summer season) or over-wintering (surviving during unfavorable winter season), is not only infected exhibiting disease symptoms but also serves as a substrate for the survival of pathogen. If the pathogen is present in the host without producing symptoms then host is known as *symptom-less carrier* and the infection is called *latent infection*. The host may be a cultivated plant (*main host*) or a wild plant of the same family (*collateral or alternative host*) or a wild plant of a different family (*alternate host*).

1. The Main Host (Cultivated Plants)

The cultivated host itself may harbour the pathogen till next season either in dormant form or in active form.

Fungi: The powdery mildew and downy mildew pathogens of grapevine survive in the infected buds till next season to serve as the primary source of inoculum.

Cucurbits are grown round the year in different parts of country as such the powdery mildew pathogen (*Erysiphe cichoracearum; Sphaerotheca fuligeana*) is continuously available in active form and the wind borne conidia can infect the crop through out the year.

Bacteria: Almost all bacterial pathogens of fruit trees survive on the host tree itself.

Ex: *Xanthomonas axonopodis* p.v. *citri* – Citrus canker.

Viruses: Viruses of crop plants survive on cultivated and weed hosts and brought back to next crop through insects.

Ex: The yellow vein mosaic virus of bhendi is available throughout the year either on bhendi or other weed hosts and is spread by white flies throughout the year.

Nematodes: Nematodes like *Meloidogyne incognitia* (root-knot nematode) have a very wide host range attacking vegetables of widely different families *viz.*, potato, tomato of Solanaceae; bhendi of Malvaceae etc. So they can find one or the other suitable host grown in rotation in the same field through out the year for active survival.

2) Collateral or Alternative Host

The pathogen may survive in active sporulating stage on wild host and from this the primary inoculum may be disseminated by wind/water/rain splashes/implements/insects to the main cultivated crops. Such hosts are referred as collateral or alternative hosts. These hosts not required for completion of the developmental cycle of the parasite. Usually these hosts belong to the related species or belong to the same family of main host. The pathogen produces the similar infective propagules on the collateral host as produced on the main host.

Ex: In the absence of the main host cucurbits, the powdery mildew pathogen and viruses of cucurbits may survive on wild cucurbits and brought back to crop through wind or insects.

3) Alternate Host

It is another host unrelated to the principal host on which a parasite can survive and different from the alternative host. Generally, alternate host is essential in completing the life cycle as in the case of heteroceous rust fungi or insect vectors that carry the viruses to the next crop season.

In the first case of alternate hosts, the completion of the life cycle to return to the aecial stage of the rust fungus is essential to infect the main host, in the absence of self-sown voluntary crop in the vicinity for infection at the start of main crop season.

In the second case, the virus is sustained by the vector till the next crop season, in the absence of self-sown voluntary crop in the vicinity for infection at the start of main crop season.

B) Saprophytic Survival Outside the Host

In the absence of cultivated host, facultative parasites/saprophytes are capable of surviving as saprophytes.

Based on the saprophytic ability, they can be divided into 3 types.

1) *Soil inhabitant:* Especially those like *Pythium, Rhizoctonia,* Sclerotia survive as soil inhabitants for considerable length of time in the absence of host plant, although in this survival resting structures like oospores, sclerotia may play a major role. The ability of such fungi to attack and colonize dead plant materials allows them to remain as active saprophytes for some time.

2) *Root inhabitant:* Vascular wilt causing fungi like *Fusarium* sp. remain in active saprophytic form only so long as the host tissues in which they are living are not completely decomposed.

3) *Rhizosphere colonizers:* Rhizosphere colonizers are the organisms which live saprophytically on dead organic matter in the Rhizosphere zone. These are slightly more tolerant to soil antagonists and usually predominant in root region that is Rhizosphere. They colonize the dead substance and survive for longer period.

Ex: Tomato leaf mold causing fungus *Cladosporium falvum.*

C) Dormant Structures in (or) on the Host (or) Outside the Host

When pathogen is unable to continue as saprophyte in plant debris (or) soil, they produce dormant structures to survive unfavorable weather (summer/winter) conditions.

Fungi: They produce resting spores. These are the structures for their inactive survival. In most of the fungal pathogens these dormant structures are the major source of survival.

1) Soil Borne Fungi

    a) Dormant spores: Clamydospores, Oospores and Perithecia

       Oospores: *Plasmopara viticola* - Downy mildew of grapes

       Clamydospores: *Fusarium oxysporium* f.sp. *cubense* – Panama wilt of Banana.

    b) Other dormant structures such as thickening of hyphae and mycelia

       Rhizomorphs: Armillaria mellea – Root rot of conifers.

2) Seed Borne Fungi

    a) Dormant mycelium or spores in true seed:

      i) Internally seed borne: The embryo or endosperm or the seed coat is infected and the parasite has parasitic relationship with the host tissues, and therefore the disease is seed borne and the seed is infected.

         Ex. Loose smut of wheat - *Ustilago tritici* – Infected embryo

         Pea seed borne mosaic virus – Seed coat (Testa)

      ii) Externally seed borne on true seed: The fungus mycelium or spores or bacterial cells are present on the surface of the seed. The seed is not infected, there being no establishment of host parasite relationship and only the pathogen is seed borne, not the disease. In fact, the seed is only infested and transports the pathogen. Sometimes the dormant structures are admixed with the seed and get entry into the field.

3) Dormant Fungal Structures on Dormant or Active Host

In addition to soil and seed, the dormant organs of fungi can also be present on the host. Thus, in downy and powdery mildew of grapevine the fungal mycelium may be present in dormant state or Oospore, or cleistothecia may be embedded in the tissues of effected organs.

4) Dormant or Active Pathogen in Vegetative Propagating Material

In vegetatively propagated crops, the infected planting material is the primary source for establishment of the pathogen in the field. Infected suckers are the main entry of fungal, viral and bacterial pathogens causing diseases in banana.

Infected bulbs stored as seed material serve as survival portal for pathogens of onion.

Bacteria: Also do not produce any resting structures and continuously live in their active parasitic stage in the living host (or) as active saprophytic stage on dead plant debris only.

Viruses: They have no resting structures and are transmitted through insects/ grafts etc.

Phanerogams: They produce seeds through which they can live in dormant stage.

Ex: *Orabanche* (broom rape) seed mixed with tobacco seed can survive for several years.

Nematodes: Majority of Nematodes survive through their dormant structures such as eggs, cysts and galls present in the soil.

Ex: Root-knot nematode, *Meloidogyne incognita* survives through eggs. Potato cyst nematode, *Globodera pallida* survives as cysts.

Dispersal of Plant Pathogens

The dispersal of the plant pathogen may occur through direct and indirect methods. Direct methods are also known as active or autonomous dispersal and indirect method as passive dispersal.

Knowledge of these methods of dispersal is essential for effective management of plant diseases to explore the possibilities of preventing dispersal and thereby breaking the infection chain.

Direct or Autonomous Dispersal

This type of dissemination is mainly responsible for spread of infection from host to host, field to field or locality to locality connected geographically very close. Autonomous dispersal of bacterial, fungi, viruses and nematodes is accomplished through A) Soil, B) Seed, and C) Plant organs.

A) Soil

As a means of autonomous dispersal can be achieved by dispersal in soil and dispersal by soil.

'*Dispersal in soil*' is by the movement of the plant pathogen in the soil under suitable conditions.

Ex: Fungi such as *Fusarium oxysporum, Sclerotium rolfsii, Armillaria mellea* can grow through mycelial elongation and reach the uninfected roots even at longer distances.

Nematodes are capable of locomotion and they move in the soil.

'*Dispersal by soil*' is by movement of soil containing the plant pathogen from one place to another.

Ex: During the cultural operations in the field, soil is moved from one place to another in the field by agricultural implements, workers or by soil erosion. Movement of farm equipment, animals from one field to another may also transport the contaminated soil and contaminate pathogen free soil with pathogens like *Sclerotium, Rizoctonia, Pythium* etc.

Another most important method of dispersal of pathogen by the soil is by transfer of soil from one place to another along with propagating materials or seedlings grown in infested soil.

Ex: Root-rot and fruit-rot of papaya caused by *Phytophthora palmivora* can spread to new plots by transplanting papaya seedlings grown in an infested field.

Ex: Dispersal or spread of root-knot disease to new fields where vegetables had not been grown earlier is mainly through seedlings raised in infested nurseries.

B) Seed

Serves as a source of autonomous dispersal since most of the cultivated crops are raised from the seeds. The transmission of diseases and transport of plant pathogen by seeds has great importance to the plant pathologists and farmers.

i) *Seed contamination*: The dormant structures of pathogen can get mixed with seed lots and get dispersed as seed contaminants.

Ex: The seed of *cuscuta* species host get mixed up during harvest of the crop.

Ex: Downy mildew fungi such as *Sclerospora* and *Personospora* produce oospores in tissue of the hosts and they may go with the seeds if not cleaned properly.

ii) *Seed transportation*: The pathogen propagules are present on seed coat without parasitic relationship with the seed.

iii) *Seed transmission*: The dormant mycelium of fungus present within the embryo of seed which is internally seed borne. There is a close contact of the pathogen with seed tissues as in wheat seed infected with loose smut pathogen.

iv) *Seed infestation*: The pathogen is present on the seed coat or in the seed lot. It is merely transport of pathogen through the seed hence the seed is infected.

v) *Seed infection*: The seed is infected only when the pathogen is present in or on it for some time and established a relationship with seed tissues. Persistence of pathogen in the seed, although seed is not viable, for many years in the form of dormant structure.

Ex: *Anguina tritici* causing ear cockle of wheat survives for 26 years in the seed, whether viable or not.

C) Autonomous Dispersal through Plant Organs or Plant Parts

This dispersal is very common in vegetatively propagated crops like sugarcane, potato, citrus, banana, etc.

Ex: Citrus tristeza is transmitted through budding and grafting.

Banana bunchy top is transmitted through Suckers.

Indirect or Passive Dispersal

This is the general and common way of dispersal of pathogens. The main agents responsible for dispersal are A) Wind; B) Water; C) Fungi; D) Insects; E) Mites; F) Nematodes; G) Other animals; and H) Man.

A) *Dissemination by Wind*

Most fungal pathogens which attack aerial parts of plant and the seeds of most parasitic plants are dispersed by air. Fungi have relatively small spores, which differ widely in their form and method of formation. Various forms of inocula in this type of pathogens are sporangia, sporangiospores, ascospores, uredospores, basidiospores and conidia etc. Spores are produced in different ways in different kind of structures. Dispersal by air occurs mainly by external forces of physical nature and thus subject is of physical rather than biological nature. Downy mildews, powdery mildews, rusts, smuts, leaf spots and sooty moulds are disseminated in this manner. Apart from spores of fungi, bits of mycelia are also disseminated by wind. In addition to this, the seeds of phanerogamic parasites and cysts of nematodes are also carried efficiently by strong wind currents.

B) *Dissemination by Water*

Water as water splash alone or in association with wind currents is an important method of liberation and dispersal of fungal spores. Coffee rust, cells of many bacteria, slimy spores of fungi like *Septoria, Fusarium* and *Colletotrichum* are dispersed by water-splash (a combination of water and air). Water itself may also be an agent of dispersal in propagules of aquatic fungi, soil-inhabiting fungi. Plant parts infected with bacteria as *Xanthomonas malvacearum* are carried by water. *Plasmodiophora brassicae* is also dispersed in this way.

Water is also important in disseminating the pathogens in three ways: (i) Bacteria, nematodes, and spores, sclerotia and fragments of mycelia present in soil are disseminated by rain or irrigation water that moves on the surface or through the soil. (ii) All bacteria and spores of many fungi are exuded in a sticky liquid and depend for their dissemination on rain; or surface or overhead irrigation water which either washes them downward or splashes them in all directions. (iii) Raindrops or drops from overhead irrigation pick up the fungal spores and bacterial cells present in the air and wash them down to land on plant surfaces.

C) *Fungi*

There are reports of about half-a-dozen viruses transmitted by fungi. The chytrid, *Olpidium brassicae* is found to transmit tobacco necrosis virus (TNV). *Olpidium* also transmits lettuce big vein (LtBV) and tobacco stunt virus (TSV). Potato virus X (PVX) is transmitted by *Synchytrium endobioticum,* and the soil borne wheat mosaic virus by *Polymyxa graminis*, potato mop-top virus by *Spongospora subterranea*.

D) *Insects*

Dispersal of fungal pathogens by insects is will-known. They feed on infected plant and move. *Ceratocystis ulmi* causing Dutch elm disease grows within eggs and carried by the beetles (*Scolytus*); sticky pycnospores of *Endothia parasitica* by insects, birds etc.

Insects, particularly aphids and leafhoppers, are the most important vectors of viruses and mycoplasma.

Ex: Banana bunchy top by the aphid, *Pentalonia nigronervosa*

Tomato spotted wilt by thrips, *Thrips tabaci*

Brinjal little leaf phytoplasma by leafhopper, *Hishimonus phycitis*

Among bacteria, which may be carried externally or internally on insects are *Erwinia amylovora* causing fire blight of pear and apple carried by flies, aphids, ants, beetles, wasps and bees; *Xanthomonas stewarti* causing bacterial blight of maize by flea beetles; *Pseudomonas savastoni* causing olive knot by olive fly.

E) Mites

Some viruses are disseminated by mites. *Nigrospora oryzae* causing wheat diseases is carried by a mite, *Pediculopsis*. *Fusarium* and *Sporotrichum* are also seen associated with mites.

They carry some viruses like pigeon pea sterility mosaic virus internally; and bacteria and spores of some fungal pathogens like *Fusarium moniliforme* var. *subglutinans* causing mango malformation externally.

F) Nematodes

Some viruses, bacteria and fungal pathogens are carried by nematodes. The nematodes carry the pathogens internally as well as externally.

Ex: Corynebacterium fascines, pathogen responsible for leafy galls of herbs is carried by ecto-parasitic nematode, *Aphelenchoides*. *Dilophospora alopeuri* is carried by *Anguina tritici*; *Fusarium oxysporum vasinfectum* causing cotton wilt by root-knot nematodes.

G) Other Animals

Some small or large animals while moving through the crop area and touching the infected plant carry the pathogens. Conidia of *Mycosphaerella linorum* can be carried by spiders, mice, frogs, birds, dogs which move on wet plants. Wood peckers carry spores of tree pathogens.

H) Man

Man is an important agent responsible for dispersal within crop area (local/regional), within the land mass (continental dispersal) or between land masses (inter-continental) dispersal. Within field it occurs through handling, through contaminated tools, through transport of contaminated soil on feet, equipment etc. Following are some examples of pathogens introduced by man.

Striga asiatica (root parasite of maize, sorghum and other cereals) was introduced in U.S.A. through seeds imported from Asia or Africa. *Endothia parasitica* (chestnut blight) was brought in from the Orient. The coffee rust (*Hemileia vastatrix*) present in Africa and Asia was introduced on coffee in Brazil. *Phytophthora infestans, Uncinula necator, Plasmopora viticola, Puccinia polyspora* and *Pseudoperonospora humuli* have spread from the New to Old world. Despite much inspection and quarantine measures, several pathogens have entered in different countries through man.

15

Epidemiology and Forecasting of Plant Diseases

Epidemics and Components of an Epidemic

An epidemic (derived from *Greek*, '*epi-*' means '*upon*'; '*-demos*' means '*people*') has been defined as "any increase of disease in a population". When a pathogen spreads to and affects many individuals within a population over an extensive area and within a relatively short time, the phenomenon is called an epidemic. A plant disease epidemic (or epiphytotic) implies the development and rapid spread of a disease on a particular kind of crop plant cultivated over a large area, a large field, a valley, a section of a country, the whole country or even a part of a continent. The study of epidemics and the factors that influence them is called **epidemiology**. Plant disease epidemics are referred as **epiphytotics.**

Plant disease epidemics develop as a result of the timely combination of the same components that result in a plant disease: susceptible population of **host** plant, a virulent **pathogen,** and favourable **environmental conditions** over fairly a long period of **time.** Besides, human activities may also help initiation and development of epidemics. When susceptible host population and virulent pathogen are juxtaposed, the duration of all favorable environmental conditions is **prolonged,** with no human intervention; the disease assumes an epidemic state.

Measurement of Plant Disease Epidemics (Epiphytotics)

Under favorable conditions, pathogens multiply and spread through populations of susceptible plants, sometimes causing extensive outbreaks of diseases. On the basis of the mode of multiplication of pathogen, the diseases may be of two types: simple interest disease and compound interest disease.

1. Simple Interest Disease

Many pathogens do not spread from plant to plant during the growing season of crop. There is only one generation of the pathogen in the crop season. The number of infected plants may increase as the season progresses but these represent new infections from primary source of inocula, rather than spread from one plant to another. This situation occurs when the pathogen does not produce secondary inoculum that otherwise can spread fast during the crop season. This denotes a disease whose increase is mathematically analogous to simple interest in money. Such pathogens include soil borne fungi attacking roots and seed, soil borne smuts infecting seedlings, etc.

2. Compound Interest Disease

Some pathogens, however, spread from plant to plant during the crop season. This denotes a disease whose increase is mathematically analogous to compound interest in money. The propagules or spores of pathogen are produced which are disseminated and infect other plants in which it, in turn, produces spores which are disseminated and infect further plants, and so on. There are several generations of pathogen in the life of crop as the pathogen repeatedly produces secondary inoculum within one crop season. Many destructive diseases like potato late blight and black stem rust of wheat belong to this category.

Structure of an Epidemic

Epidemic develops as a consequence of the interactions of the populations of their two components, **host** and **pathogen,** as influenced by **environmental** and **human** interference over time. The interactions of host and pathogen produce the third component, **disease.** Each of the three primary components (host, pathogen, and disease) consists of sub-components. The sub-components for host are a) seasonal/annual/perennial/tree; b) its growth stages *viz.*, seedling, tillering, blossoming; c) method of propagation *viz.*, seed/vegetative; d) reaction to the pathogen *viz.*, resistant/susceptible. Sub-components for the pathogen are a) pathogenicity *viz.*, virulent/avirulent; b) host specificity *viz.*, varietal specialization/race; c) nature of sporulation *viz.*, kind and amount of inoculum; d) dispersal *viz.*, wind, water, vector; and e) survival *viz.*, duration and form). Sub-components for disease include a) infection type and nature *viz.*, no. of lesions, size, rate, systemic, localized; b) pathogenesis *viz.*, incubation period; c) spread (infection gradient in plant population); d) rate of multiplication *viz.*, length of reproduction cycle, duration, number of cycles per season; and e) survival period *viz.*, longevity in days/months/years.

Development of an Epidemic

For a disease to spread over large area and develop into an epidemic, the right **combinations** of environmental factors must occur and spread constantly or repeatedly at frequent intervals over a large area. A disease can occur in a garden, a green house or a small field, but it takes an **epidemic** form when the disease develops and spreads rapidly on a particular kind of crop plant cultivated over a large area *viz.*, a large field, a valley, part of a country, the whole country or even part of a continent. Therefore, the **first** component of a plant disease epidemic is a large area planted with a more or less genetically uniform single crop plant in fields being close together. The **second** component of an epidemic is the presence or appearance of a virulent pathogen at some point of the active growing season among or near the cultivated host plants, *i.e.*, cohabitations of host plants and pathogens. Such cohabitation may occur daily. But an epidemic will develop only when the combination and progression of right environmental conditions exist. The **third** component of epidemic is this combination of environmental factors. Epidemics develop only when the combination and progression of the right **sets** of environmental conditions, *i.e.*, moisture, temperature and wind or insect vector, coincide with the susceptible stages of the plant and with the production of viable inoculum, its spread, inoculation, penetration, infection, and reproduction of the pathogen. Lastly, and the most important **fourth** component of an epidemic is that in each new location, the same set of environmental factors must be **repeated** so that new infections, reproduction and dispersal of pathogen must occur as quickly as possible. These conditions must be repeated several times within each location. It is these repeated several infections that would result in more or less complete destruction of almost every plant within the area of an epidemic. Fortunately, these conditions do not occur very often over very large areas, as such plant epidemics are relatively rare.

Briefly, we may say that the following conditions favour the epiphytotics: (i) virulent pathogen with short sporulation (latent) period, (ii) rapid spore germination and infection, (iii) susceptible plant at susceptible stage of growth, (iv) intensive monoculture of susceptible plants over large areas, and (v) environmental conditions favourable to the pathogen at all points in the infections cycle, *i.e.*, sporulation and subsequent liberation, dissemination and deposition of spores in viable form, germination, infection and growth in host tissues. Weather during the intercrop period as well as during crop season can be important in seasonal carry-over and it may affect the initial outbreak and subsequent spread of the pathogen.

Modeling and Computer Simulation of Epidemics

In recent years, attempts have been made to develop models of potential epidemics of some common and severe diseases. Various components and sub-components of the disease are taken into account in quantitative terms to construct a model.

The availability of computers has allowed us to write programmes that allow simulation of epidemics of several plant diseases. **EPIDEM,** was the first computer simulation programme written in 1969 for early blight epidemics of potato and tomato caused by *Alternaria solani*. This resulted from modeling each stage of the life cycle of the fungus. Subsequently such programmes were written for *Mycosphaerella* blight of chrysanthemums (**MYCOS**), southern corn leaf blight caused by *Helminthosporium maydis* (**EPICORN)**, and apple scab caused by *Venturia inaequalis* (**EPIVEN)**. **EPIDEMIC** was also written for stripe rust of wheat. In computer simulation, the dates describing the various sub-components of the epidemic and control methods at specific points are given to the computer.

With the success of modeling and computer simulation, we could be able to **forecast plant disease epidemics.** Forecast is extremely useful to farmers in the practical management of crop diseases.

16

Principles of
Plant Disease Management

Measures taken to prevent incidence of a disease, reduce the amount of inoculum, that initiates and spreads the disease and finally minimize the loss caused by the disease have traditionally been called as control measures. Now, the word control has been substituted with management. Actually control denotes permanent settlement of the problem. No plant disease can be permanently controlled. The disease can only be managed so that the loss can be kept below economic damage level. Thus management conveys the concept of a continuous process and is based not only on the principles of eradication of pathogen but also on the principles of maintaining the damage. The plant disease management is based on the following principles.

1) Avoidance of the Pathogen

The aim of this method is to make the host not to come in contact with the pathogen and to see that susceptible stage of the host and favourable conditions for the pathogen should not coincide. This can be achieved by:

A) Proper Selection of Field

Successful cultivation of a crop depends to a great extent on selection of proper field. Generally, it is not advisable to grow the crop in the same field year after year. If the same crop is grown in the same field, there is a chance of build-up of inoculum in the seed and the disease becomes severe in the future years.

Ex: The soil-borne diseases like Panama wilt in banana (*Fusarium oxysporium* f.sp. *cubense*) can be avoided by not growing the same crop in the same field every year.

B) Selection of Pathogen-Free Propagation Materials and Seed

Many diseases are introduced into the crop only through seed (or) other propagating material like suckers, bulbs, tubers, cuttings, etc. Such diseases can be easily controlled by selecting pathogen-free seed or propagating material from disease-free areas.

Ex: Planting of such pathogen-free seed in a field is often most efficient method of control of certain diseases like loose smut of wheat with pathogen-free seed, red-rot of sugarcane with pathogen-free sets, banana suckers from crop free of bunchy top disease etc.

C) Choice of Time of Sowing

In many diseases, the incidence is most serve when the susceptible stage of plant growth and favourable conditions for the pathogen coincides. While choosing the time of sowing, it should be taken into consideration that susceptible stage of plant growth and other environmental conditions favourable for pathogen activity do not fall at the same time. Alternation in date of sowing can help in avoidance of favourable conditions for pathogens.

Ex: Pea planted soon after rains, where soil temperature and moisture are at a high level, show high incidence of root-rot (*Macrophomina phaseolina*). Late sowing, *i.e.*, sowing during November-December helps in saving the crop because of low soil temperature.

D) Disease Escaping Varieties

Certain varieties of crop plants escape disease because of their growth character like early maturing or late maturing varieties.

Ex: Varieties of pea which mature early (by January) escape powdery mildew caused by *Erysiphe polygoni*. This incidence generally becomes serious in varieties maturing late after January.

2) Exclusion of Inoculum

It is designed to keep the pathogen away from entering the area in which host is growing *i.e.*, it aims at limiting the spread of the pathogen from the one region to the other. This can be achieve by:

A) Quarantine Regulations

Quarantine can be defined as legal restriction of movement of agricultural conditions from one place to another for the purpose of prevention of introduction of pests and diseases in uninfected area. These regulations are effective in preventing the movement of dormant structures of pathogens from one place to other through plant and planting material. The quarantine laws were first formulated in U.S.A. in 1912 under Federal Quarantine Act. Quarantine regulations are of three types:

i) Domestic/National quarantine

ii) Foreign/International quarantine

iii) Total embargo

i) Domestic/National Quarantine

Movement of insects, pathogens and their hosts is restricted from one state to another within the country. These regulations are aimed at preventing the introduction of diseases from infected areas to non-infected areas.

Ex: Domestic quarantine exists in India against Banana bunchy top disease. The movement of any part of banana including suckers stems and leaf material used for planting except fruit is prohibited from Kerala, Assam, Bihar, Orissa, and West Bengal.

ii) Foreign/International Quarantine

Movement of insects, pathogens and their hosts is restricted from one country to the other. The planting material should be imported only through prescribed ports of entry.

Ex: Air ports – Mumbai, Chennai, Vizag. Inspite of strict quarantine regulations some of the serious plant diseases were introduced from one country to the other.

Phytopthora infestans introduced from S. America to Europe in 1830.

Coffee rust was introduced from Sri Lanka into India in 1879.

iii) Total Embargo

It is the total ban on the import of a specific host plant from specific area.

Ex: Total ban on import of Spanish chestnut plants into Britain to prevent entry of chestnut blight pathogen, *Endothia parasitica*.

B) Phytosanitary Certificate

It is an official certificate from the country of origin of seed or planting material which should accompany the consignment. It is an essential requirement to import seed or planting material without which the material may be refused entry.

C) Inspection and Seed Certificate

Certain crops are grown exclusively for seed purpose. Such crops are periodically inspected for the presence of seed-borne diseases and necessary precautions are taken to remove the diseased plants. The crop is then certified as disease-free. This practice helps to prevent inter-and intra-regional spread of seed-borne diseases.

3) Eradication

It aims at elimination of the pathogen from an infected area by destruction of primary and secondary source of inoculums thus breaking the infection chain. If a pathogen enters an area in spite of above precautions, the eradication procedures are adopted.

Eradication Involves

A) Rouging

It involves the removal and destruction of infected plants or plant parts from the field in an early stage of disease. It prevents spread of disease to healthy plants and also ensures healthy seed.

Ex: Rouging of infected area heads prevents the spread of disease to healthy flowers, citrus canker (*X. axonopodis* p.v. *citri*)

B) Eradication of Alternate and Collateral Host

Alternate host: It is the host belonging to the family different from that of main host which is helpful in the completion of life cycle of the pathogen.

Collateral host: It is the host belonging to the same family of the main host which is helpful in perpetuation of pathogens.

C) Cultural Practices

For development of a disease, the contact between host and pathogen must occur in environment favorable to the pathogen. Suitable adjustments in cultural practices can modify the environment, making it unfavorable for pathogen and disease development. These practices reduce the density and activity of the inoculum. Such practices include crop rotation, green manuring, deep ploughing etc.

Ex: Crop Rotation: It is growing of different unrelated crops in a field in a pre-planned succession. If the same or related crop is grown continuously year after year, the inoculum of the pathogen builds up in the soil. After a few years the disease becomes severe and the crop cannot be grown.

If crop rotation is followed with other crops which are non-hosts for the pathogen, the disease can be minimized. This is an old practice by which sources of primary inoculum are eradicated. Soil pathogens which survive only on the living host as long as the host residue persists as substrata for their survival can be completely eradicated by crop rotation. Soil-borne pathogens with narrow host range can be reduced in the soil by planting the plants belonging to the species not attacked by the particular pathogen for 3-4 years. The principle involved in this method is starvation of the pathogen due to continuous absence of their living host.

Ex: A crop rotation sequence of wheat-oat followed by potato-onion-maize is recommended for potato against common scab caused by *Streptomyces scabies*.

D) Biological Control (or) Bio-Control

It is defined as any practice whereby survival and activity of a pathogen is reduced through the agency of any other living organism with the result that there is a reduction in the incidence of the disease caused by the pathogen. This method aims at either direct protection of plants from pathogen (or) at eradication (or) reduction of inoculum by using antagonistic organisms, mostly micro-organisms. A few biological methods also aim at improving the plant resistance. Ex: Systemic acquired resistance.

The recognized general mechanisms of biological control are competition, antibiosis, parasitism and predation. The major microbial metabolites involved in disease suppression by bio-control agents include antibiotics, ammonia, enzymes, hydrogen cyanide etc. Interest in biological control, in fact, first arose in 1920s when some plant pathogens could be suppressed by introduction of some naturally occurring antibiotic-producing microbes.

☆ In recent years, the increasing information on hazardous effects of synthetic chemicals on plants and animal health have alarmed the scientists to seek an alternate method like biological control, which should not cause pollution and should be non-phytotoxic.

☆ Biological control practices for direct protection involve the deployment of antagonistic micro-organisms at the infection court before (or) immediately after infection. There are several cases of successful biological control, only for soil-borne diseases and hardly a few are registered for commercial use. Several antagonistic fungi and bacteria have been used as bio-control agents against a number of soil-borne diseases caused by *Pythium, Phytophthora, Sclerotium, Rhizoctonia, Fusarium, Meloidogyne, Agrobacterium* which can be applied to the seed (or) as soil application.

Some examples of fungal bio-control agents and their commercial preparations:

i) *Trichoderma Viride*

ii) *T. harziancium*

iii) *Gliocladium Virens*

iv) *Glomus fasciculatum* (Endomycorrhizal fungi)

Some examples of bacterial bio-control agents:

i) *Agrobacterium radiobacter* strain K-84 against *A. tumefaciens* - Galltrol

ii) *Pseudomonas flouroscens*- Dagger–G

iii) *Bacillus subtilis*-Kodiak

E) Physical Methods

The physical agents most commonly used in controlling plant diseases are temperature, use of plastic coverings, etc.

i) Soil Solarization

It is a method of heating soil by covering it with transparent polythene sheeting during hot periods to control soil-borne diseases. The technique has been commercially exploited for growing high value crops in diseased soils in environments with hot summer, regularly exceeding 35°C. It is the most advanced field technology for control of soil-borne diseases which include control of *Fusarium* wilts in vegetable crops. The major benefits of soil solarization are reduction of soil-borne pathogens, control of weeds, insects pests, release of plant nutrients etc. Soil solarization is based on trapping solar Infra-Red radiation by tightly covering the soil with clear polythene sheet of 400 gauge (100 micrometers thick) for several weeks during hot summer months. This results in a significant increase of soil temperature [10°-15°C above normal depending on the soil depth] up to a point where most pathogens are vulnerable to heat effects.

ii) Hot Water Treatment

Hot water treatment of certain seeds, bulbs, nursery stock and other planting material is used to kill any pathogen which they carry externally or internally without loosing viability of the material.

Ex: *Alternaria brassicae* from cabbage seeds can be eliminated successfully by using hot water treatment. For powdery mildew of beans, the seed is kept in hot water at 43-50°C for 20 min. to reduce the disease.

4) Protection

Protection is one of the most commonly used methods of controlling plant diseases in the field, greenhouses and storage. This is achieved through the use of chemicals in plant disease management by creating a toxic barrier between the host surface and the pathogen. In the process the pathogen is eradicated from a particular site on the host. According to the nature of the pathogen against which the anti-pathogen chemical is used, the chemical is generally called as fungicide (against fungi) or bactericide (against bacteria) or nematicide (against nematode) or weedicide (against weed) etc.

A) Fungicides

A fungicide is an agent that kills (or) inhibits the development of fungal spore (or) mycelium.

Classification of Fugicides

According to the mode of their action, the fungicides can be grouped into the following categories.

I. Protectants

Chemicals which are effective only when used before infection by the pathogen are known as protectants. These chemicals may be contact protective fungicides (which kill the pathogen when it comes in contact with the host) or residual protective fungicides (established as a fixed layer on the surface of the host by spraying, dusting, etc., and destroy the pathogen when it lands on the host). These are applied as prophylactic measures and are non-systemic in action.

Ex: Zineb, sulphur, captan, thiram etc.

II. Eradicants

These are the chemicals which can eradicate the dormant (or) active pathogen from the host surface in which infection could possibly occur. They can remain effective on or in the host for some time and function as protectant also.

Ex: Lime sulphur.

III. Therapeutants

A therapeutant is an agent that inhibits the development of a disease in a plant when applied after infection by a pathogen, thereby curing the plant. Mostly chemotherapeutants are systemic. They enter the host and effect the deep-seated pathogen and is fungistatic (preventing the sporulation) in action.

Ex: plantavax, aureofungin, carbendazim.

IV. Systemic Fungicides

A systemic fungicide is one which gets translocated from the point of application and acts on the pathogen at other parts of the plant. This can eradicate established infection and protects new parts of the plant.

Ex: Oxycarboxin, benomyl, carbendazim, carboxin

According to the method of use, fungicides are classified into:-

  i) *Seed protectants*: Captan, Thiram

  ii) *Soil fumigants (pre-plant)*: Formaldehyde, Vapam

  iii) *Foliage protectants*: Captan, Zineb (growing plants)

  iv) *Soil fungicides*: Captan, Thiram

  v) *Fruit protectants*: Captan, Maneb

  vi) *Tree wound dressing fungicides*: Bordeaux paste

  vii) *Antibiotics*: These are substances produced by micro organisms which in very dilute concentrations have the capacity to inhibit the growth of other microorganisms. Most antibiotics are toxic to bacteria, mollicutes and fungi.

  a) Streptomycin: Produced from *Streptomyces griseus* and sold as Agrimycin effective against fire blight of apple, citrus canker.

  b) Tetracycline: Produced from *Streptomyces rimosus* and sold as terramycin used against bacteria and mollicutes.

  c) Cycloheximide: Produced from *Streptomyces griseus* and sold as Actidione used against powdery mildew of beans, stem rust of wheat.

  d) Griseofulvin: Isolated from *Pencillium griso-fulvum* found effective against powdery mildew of cucurbits, downy mildew of cucurbits.

  e) Aureofungin: Isolated from *Streptomyces cinnamomeus* var. *terricola* commercially marketed by Hindustan Antibiotics Ltd. Pimpre (Pune) effective against rice blast, damping off disease of vegetables, ganoderma root-rot of coconut.

Formulation of Fungicides and Method of Application

Commercial fungicides are formulated in various ways. Most commonly available formulations are dusts, water dispersible powders, emulsifiable concentrates, suspensions (or) slurries. These fungicides are applied as seed treatments, soil application, foliar spraying, dusting, paste applications or fumigants etc.

B) Bactericides

Any chemical compound that kills or inhibits the bacteria is called Bactericide. Most antibiotics are toxic to bacteria, mollicutes, and fastidious vascular bacteria. The most important antibiotics used against bacterial diseases are Streptomycin, Tetracyclin, Cycloheximide. They are used to control these pathogens causing spots, blights, rusts, fire blight etc.

C) Nematicides

A chemical compound that kills the nematodes. Many of the nematicides have broad spectrum and are volatile soil fumigants active against not only nematodes but also insects, fungi, bacteria and weeds.

Types of Nematicides

Nematicides in commercial use basically belong to:

i) Fumigants

Halogenated hydrocarbons and isothiocyanate; Gas, volatile liquid (or) solids that diffuse through the soil pore spaces as a vapour. They are dissolved and dispersed in soil moisture to kill nematode larvae. These are not very specific and used for control of many nematodes, soil insects, fungal and bacterial plant pathogens.

Ex: Halogenated hydrocarbons – methyl bromide (Meth-O – gas); Chloropicrin (tear gas)

Sodium methyl dithiocarbamate – Metam sodium; Vapam.

ii) Non-fumigants

These compounds belong to Organo-phosphates and carbonates. These are contact and systemic nematicides. They have little fumigant action and do not kill the nematodes directly. These are non-volatile and non-fumigant nematicides, relatively less phytotoxic and can be applied before (or) at the time of planting (or) even on standing crop.

Ex: Organophosphates – phorate (Thimet); phenomiphos (Nemacus); carbofuran (Furadon)

5) Disease Resistance (Immunization)

Though there is no antibody producing system in plants, treatment with pathogens sometimes leads to disease resistance. Besides, genetic resistance of the host can also be improved by breeding for disease resistance.

A) Induced Resistance/Systemic Acquired Resistance

Inoculation of plants with certain pathogens often leads to temporary (or) permanent immunization of the plants *i.e.*, induced resistance to a pathogen to which the host plant is normally susceptible. Resistance generated in a plant by treatments involving different pathogens is called induced or systemic acquired resistance. There are many examples in which plants infected with one pathogen become more resistant to subsequent infection by another pathogen.

Ex: Bean and sugar beet inoculated with viruses show greater resistance to some obligate fungal pathogens causing rusts, powdery mildew. In tobacco mosaic virus infection induces a systemic resistance not only to the virus itself but also to *Phytopthora parasitica* var. *nicotinae* and *Pseudomonas tabaci*.

B) Resistant Varieties

Resistance is the ability of a host plant to suppress (or) retard the activity of a pathogen (or) other injury factor. The use of resistant varieties is the least expensive, most safe and most effective means of controlling plant diseases in crops.

Advantages of Resistant Varieties

1. The use of resistant variety is the simplest, practical, effective and economical method of plant disease control.

2. Resistant variety not only offers protection against disease, but can also save time and money spent on other control measures.

3. For certain diseases like viral and vascular wilts for which suitable chemical control is not available, use of resistant varieties is the only practical method of control.

4. Resistant varieties do not pollute the environment and are not toxic to man and livestock.

5. Resistant varieties are effective only against target organisms and do not harm beneficial organisms like hyperparasites of the pathogen.

   Ex: Mango variety *Manjira* is resistant to Powdery mildew.

   Banana variety *Vamanakeli* is resistant to Panama wilt.

17
Integrated Plant Disease Management

Integrated disease management (IDM) is an approach that attempts to prevent pathogens from causing economic crop losses by using a variety of management methods that are cost effective and cause least damage to the environment. The use of different methods like suitable cultural practices, resistant varieties, bio-control agents coupled with minimal use of chemicals is the only answer for the management of all the diseases affecting a crop as no single method can give an effective and economical control of any crop disease for a longer period.

The main goals of IDM are:

1. To eliminate (or) reduce initial inoculums.
2. To reduce the effectiveness of initial inoculums.
3. To increase the resistance of the host.
4. To delay the onset of disease.

An integrated disease management program can be developed against any disease affecting any crop. Some examples of successful use of integrated diseases are:

Ex: 1. Potato

Early blight (*Alternaria solani*), late blight (*P. infestans*) black scurf (*R. solani*), wilt Raltsonia (*Pscudomonas solanaceaurm*), Root-knot (*Meloidogyne incognita*), Golden Nematode (*Globadera mustochiensis*) mosaic diseases are the quite common diseases affecting potato. Due to the vegetative nature of propagation, all the diseases are primarily seed (tuber) borne and some of them are soil borne too. Disease spread by soil, insects, water and wind is common. Therefore, the crop improvement in quality and quantity of yields through integrated disease management can be brought about by adopting a schedule prepared on the following lines.

A) Cultural Practices

1) Proper Selection of Field

Seed tubers must be planted in a field without early history of disease incidence or free from old tubers which may harbour some of the pathogens. The land must have proper drainage and high fertility.

2) Use of Healthy Planting Stock

Since tubers are the main source of introduction of pathogens in the field, tubers certified free from disease must be used for planting. Alternatively, tubers collected from disease-free plants may be used to keep the tubers free from the entire tuber borne pathogens. Additional precautions can be taken by treating the seed tubers with fungicides such as benomyl. The chemical treatment helps in eradication of residual inoculum from seed and protects it during germination, emergence and further development.

B) Use of Resistant Varieties

In areas where late blight regularly occurs every year it is always advisable to grow only Kurfi Naveen, Kufri Jeevan etc.

Resistant Varieties

Variety	Resistant/Immune to following Diseases
Kufri Anand, Kufri Giriraj, Kufri Chipsona-1, Kufri Chipsona-2, Kufri Jawahar, Kufri Sutlej	Resistant to late blight
Kufri Swarna	Resistant to late blight and Cyst nematode
Kufri Sherpa	Resistant to late blight and Wart
Kufri Badshah	Resistant to both late and early blights and PVX
Kufri Naveen	Immune to Wart
Kufri Muthu	Resistant to late blight

C) Date of Planting

Date of planting should be decided according to prevailing soil temperature and moisture to prevent periods favorable to the disease.

D) Crop Rotation

The crop may be rotated with legumes (or) corn which is non-hosts to many potato pathogens.

E) Eradication of Collateral and Self-Sown Crop

Many fungal, bacterial and viral diseases are retained throughout the year on such plants serving as reservoirs of primary inoculum. Destruction of these reservoirs by the onset of next season is essential.

F) Destruction

Prompt disposal of discarded potato seed tubers and crop residue by destruction also helps in production of healthy crop.

G) Rouging

Plants showing viral infections should promptly be removed and destroyed throughout the season as soon as the symptoms are noticed.

H) Chemical Sprays

Regular sprayings with fungicides such as zineb, mancozeb, etc., at regular intervals should be done to prevent late and early blight.

I) Vector Control

Potato crop suffers from several viruses which are transmitted by vectors like aphids. Regular monitoring and chemical sprays suitable against vectors must be done.

J) Care by Workers

The workers should follow sanitary precautions to prevent entry and spread of diseases during the field operations. Damage to tubers while harvesting should be minimized to avoid storage loss and infection of tubers during storage.

Ex: 2. Banana

Banana is a crop that is propagated vegetatively through suckers. All banana diseases occurring in the field can be transmitted by disease suckers and make entry into new areas of cultivation. Diseases like bunchy top entered this country through propagating material from other countries. Therefore, cultural methods are foremost in avoiding and exclusion of the pathogens that are endemic or may be present in areas from which the planting material is supplied. The general integrated management practices covering all important diseases are listed below from which necessary steps as required for the region or area or diseases can be followed.

   ☆ The first and foremost precaution to avoid entry of any pathogen into the crop is to select proper healthy planting material by personally inspecting the mother garden two-to-four times during the season to ascertain the disease incidence in it before obtaining the suckers.

   ☆ Never depend on others like brokers, commission agents and commercial suppliers for supply of planting material.

   ☆ Quarantine and exclusion procedures by restricting the movement of corms, suckers and soil that could be carrying the pathogens are the most effective means to control the diseases.

☆ Planting material free of the pathogen and propagated in accredited tissue culture laboratories should be used.

☆ Growing of paddy followed by banana for 3-5 years once or twice, use of quick lime near the base of the plant and soaking with water and avoiding sunflower or sugarcane in crop rotation helps to reduce the disease incidence of panama wilt in endemic areas.

☆ Moko disease can be minimised by exposing soil to sunlight.

☆ Flooding the panama wilt infested field for 2 to 6 months helps in reducing the disease.

☆ Application of bioagents, such as, *Trichoderma viride* or *Pseudomonas fluorescence* in the soil is effective in managing soil borne pathogens.

☆ Soil drench with vapam (metham sodium) @ 850 g per 100 litres of water.

☆ Dipping of suckers in 0.1 per cent Carbendazim (10g/10 litres of water) followed by bimonthly drenching starting from 6 months after planting is also recommended to control fungal infections carried through rhizomes.

☆ Soil drenching with bleaching powder was found beneficial in checking bacterial soft rot.

☆ Treating suckers at 40°C with dry heat for 1 day followed by treatment with 120 ppm aureofungin can minimize infectious chlorosis.

☆ Use of tissue culture grown plantlets reduces the risk of disease transmission through suckers. However, banana streak virus (BSV) can be carried *in vitro* plantlets, as it is not eliminated by shoot-tip culture. Hence, parts of leaves with pronounced BSV symptoms should be used for serological indexing.

☆ Highly infected soil should not be replanted with banana for at least 3-4 years.

☆ Early detection and immediate eradication of infected plants. The diseased plants along with rhizomes should be destroyed as soon as they are detected.

☆ Disinfecting cutting knives and providing better drainage.

☆ Before the onset of the warm, rainy season, all sigatoka-affected leaves must be removed from the plant to reduce the inoculum.

☆ Spraying of bunches/plants with 0.1 per cent carbendazim or thiophanate methyl or propiconazole or 0.2 per cent chlorothalonil at 15-20 days intervals is quite effective against sigatoka and anthracnose diseases. The last spray should be given 15-20 days before harvesting. Remove and destroy trash including severely infected leaves and bunches before spraying.

☆ Spray 1 per cent Bordeaux mixture or 0.3 per cent copper oxy chloride twice or thrice at 7-10 days interval if freckle leaf spot incidence is noticed.

☆ The aphids should be controlled to check disease spread of viral diseases by spraying with 0.5 per cent Metasystox or 0.2 per cent Dimethoate.

☆ Placing a polythene bag over the stem before the hands emerged and removal of the pistil and perianth by hand as soon as the fingers emerged were effective to manage cigar end rot.

☆ Herbicides, *e.g.*, Fernoxone; 2, 4-D and 2, 4, 5-T can be used to kill infected plants *in situ* and dieldrin sprayed onto a chopped down mat will prevent insects transmitting diseases to the unaffected plants.

☆ As flower visiting insects are main agents for transmitting moko disease the practice of removing the bud from the male axis before the bunch matures reduces the incidence.

☆ Harvest fruit at the correct stage of maturity as fruit harvested too young are more susceptible to crown rot and thiabendazole applied as a dip treatment @ 200 ppm a.i. after harvest controls any latent infection.

☆ Avoiding susceptible varieties and growing resistant ones.

Disease	Susceptible Varieties	Resistant Varieties
Panama wilt	Amruthapani, Sirumalai and Monthan	Poovan, Moongil, Vamankeli and Bontha.Seeded bananas like *Musa balbisiana* are immune
Sigatoka leaf spot	—	Blue Java; Bluggoe; Ducasse; Gold Finger; Pisang Ceylan; Simoi
Freckle leaf spot	—	Cavendish
Infectious chlorosis	—	Karu Bale

Ex: 3. Tomato

Tomato is a versatile crop with a wide range of pathogens including fungi, bacteria, viruses and nematodes which are either air-borne, or soil-borne or seed-borne or even carried by planting material and also transmitted by vectors. The management of this crop with least disease loss is possible only when all the strategies of integrated disease management are applied. The management practices have to be selected based on the history of occurrence of diseases that are endemic or sporadic or diseases that occurred in epidemic form. Some diseases have collateral or alternative hosts or weeds grown in the season or off-season.

☆ Start with certified, disease-free seed.

☆ Heat water seed treatment at 50°C for 25 minutes.

☆ Seed treatment with captan or thiram at 3 g per kg seed.

☆ A 3 to 4 year crop rotation with non-solanaceous crops.

☆ Destruction of collateral, alternative crops and weeds.

☆ Provide good soil drainage.

☆ Seed treatment with 4 g *Trichoderma viride* formulation per kg seed is helpful in reducing the incidence southern blight.

☆ Apply a fungicidal soil drench if damping-off is a problem.

☆ Orient rows in the direction of prevailing winds, avoid shaded areas, and avoid wind barriers.

☆ Water seedlings only when the soil or growth medium is dry, preferably in the morning to allow drying to occur by the late afternoon.

☆ For seedbeds, choose well-drained locations and keep the seedbed well ventilated and dry.

☆ Avoid overcrowding of plants and the movement of infested soil or contaminated plant material into the nursery bed.

☆ Sow 5-6 rows of barrier crops like maize, jowar or bajra around main tomato field at least 2 months before transplanting seedlings in the field.

☆ Staking of plants, removal of lower foliage (upto 30 cm) and fruits helps in prevention of initiation and spread of soil-borne diseases.

☆ Promote good air circulation by proper spacing of plants.

☆ Avoid excess overhead irrigation, water plants in the late morning and avoid working when plants are wet.

☆ Remove and destroy crop residue at the end of the season or plough residues into the soil to promote breakdown by soil micro-organisms and to physically remove the spore source from the soil surface.

☆ Fertilize the crop properly as healthy plants with adequate nutrition are less susceptible to diseases.

☆ At the base of the plant affected by Sothern blight, drenching soil with Chestnut compound 3 g/l to check the spread.

☆ Spray 2-3 times with 0.05 per cent dimethoate or monocrotophos or 0.02 per cent metasystox at 10 days intervals to control vectors of viral diseases.

☆ Weekly spray of 0.25 per cent zineb or maneb or mancozeb or chlorothalonil or 0.1 per cent benomyl or carbendazim in the nursery bed and in main field help to reducing the incidence of foliar diseases.

☆ Use of resistant or tolerant varieties.

Disease	Resistant varieties
Early blight	Juliet, Old Brook, Big Beef
Fusarium and *Verticillium* wilts	Beef Master; Better Boy and Roma
Tomato mosaic	Sweet Chelsea, Sweet Million, Sweet Quartz, Shirley

Appendices

Consolidated List of Major Diseases of Horticultural Crops

Diseases of Fruit Crops

Sl.No.	Common Name	Name of the Pathogen
BANANA		
1.	Panama Wilt	*Fusarium oxysporum* f.*cubense*
2.	Anthroancnose and fruit rot	*Gloeosporium musarum*
3.	Sigatoka leaf spot	*Cercopora musae*
4.	Black tip or cigar end rot	*Deightoneilla torulosum*
5.	Freckle or Black spot	*Phyllostictina musarum*
6.	Bacterial leaf spot	*Xanthomonas campestris* pv. *musicola*
7.	Bunchy top	*Musa Virus - 1*
8.	Moko Wilt of Banana	*Ralstonia solanacearum*
9.	Infectious Chlorosis	*Cucumber mosaic virus*
MANGO		
1.	Powdery mildew	*Oidium mangiferae*
2.	Anthracnose	*Collectotrichum gloeosporioides*
3.	Grey blight	*Pestaliotiopsis mangiferae*
4.	Sooty mould	*Capnodiurm ramosum*
5.	Red rust	*Cephaleurus parasiticus*
6.	Black spot	*X.campestris* pv. *mangiferae indicae*
7.	Malformation	Virus, fungal, mites, cultural practices, nutrition deficiency and hormonal inbalance
8.	Die-Back	*Lasiodiplodia theobraomae*
9.	Canker	*Xanthomonas campestris* pv. *mangiferae indicae*
GRAPEVINE		
1.	Powdery mildew	*Uncinula necator*
2.	Downy mildew	*Plasmopara viticola*
3.	Anthracnose	*Gloeosporium ampelophagum* (imperfect stage)
4.	Bunch Rot	*Botrytis cinerea*

Sl.No.	Common Name	Name of the Pathogen
CITRUS		
1.	Leaf fall and fruit rot	*Phytophthorn palmivora*
2.	Die-back or wither tip	*Colletotrichum gloeosoporioides*
3.	Powdery mildew	*Oidium tingitanium*
4.	Sooty mould	*Capnodium citri*
5.	Canker	*Xanthomonas campestris* pv. *citri*
6.	Red rust	*Cephaleurous parasiticus*
7.	Ring spot	Citrus ring spot virus (CRSV)
8.	Greening	Rickettsia Like Organism (RLO's)
9.	Tristeza or quick decline	Virus
10.	Deficiency diseases	Zinc, Magnesium, Boron and Manganese
GUAVA		
1.	Anthracnose or fruit rot	*Gloeosporium psidii*
2.	Sooty mould	*Meliola* sp.
3.	Red rust	*Cephaleuros parasiticus*
4.	Wilt	*Fusarium oxysporum* f.sp. *psidii, Macrophomina phaseolina* and *F.solanii*
SAPOTA		
1.	Leaf spot	*Phavopleospora indica*
2.	Sooty mould	*Capnodium* spp.
PAPAYA		
1.	Foot rot	*Pythium butleri*
2.	Leaf spot	*Phyllosticta sawata*
3.	Dry root rot	*Macrophomina phaseolina*
4.	Mosaic	Papaya mosaic virus
5.	Leaf curl	Papaya leaf curl virus
JACK		
1.	Fruit rot	*Rhizopus artocarpi*
2.	Leaf spot	*Colletotrichum lagenarium*
PINEAPPLE		
1.	Leaf and fruit rot	*Ceratocystis paradoxa*
2.	Root rot	*Phytophthora parasitica*
3.	Wilt	Pine apple wilt virus

Sl.No.	Common Name	Name of the Pathogen
BER		
1.	Powdery mildew	*Oidium* sp.*Oidiopsis* sp.
2.	Leaf spot	*Cercospora* sp.
APPLE		
1.	Scab	*Ventuira inaequlis*
2.	Powdery mildew	*Podosphaera leucotricha*
3.	Fire blight	*Erwinia amylovora*
4.	Crown gall	*Agrabacterium tumefacients*
3.	Pink desease	*Corticium salmonicolor*
4.	Mosaic	Apple mosaic virus
5.	Dapple apple	Viroid
6.	Apple Scar skin	Viroid like RNA
PEACH		
1.	Leaf curl	*Taphrina deformans*
2.	Powdery mildew	*Sphaerotheca apnnos*
PLUM		
1.	Brown rot	*Sclerotinia fructigena*
STRAWBERRY		
1.	Powdery Mildew	*Sphaerotheca macularis* f.sp *fragariae*
2.	Verticillium Wilt	*Verticillium dahliae*
STONE FRUITS		
1.	Leaf Curl	*Taphrina deformans*
2.	Brown Rot	*Monilinia fructicola, M. fructigena*

Diseases of Vegetable Crops

Sl.No.	Common Name	Name of the Pathogen
TOMATO		
1.	Damping off	*Pythium aphanidermatum*
2.	Early blight	*Alternaria solani*
3.	Wilt	*Fusarium oxysporum* f.sp.*lycopersici*
4.	Mosaic	Tomato mosaic virus (ToMV) Tobamo virus
5.	Leaf curl	*Tobacco leaf curl*, bigemini virus

Sl.No.	Common Name	Name of the Pathogen
6.	Spotted witlt	Tomato spotted wilt virus (TSWV) Tospovirus
7.	Bacterial canker	*Zanthomonas campestric* pv. *vesicatoria*
8.	Shoe-string	Potato virus Y

BHENDI

1.	Powdery mildew	*Erysiphe communis*
2.	Leaf spot	*Cercospora malayensis*
3.	Vein clearing or yellow vein mosaic	Bigemini virus (YVMV)

BRINJAL

1.	Leaf spot or blight	*Alternaria solani*
2.	Little leaf	*Phytoplasma*
3.	Aecial stage of bajra rust	*Puccinia penniseti*
4.	Damping off	*Pythium aphanidermatum*
5.	Phomopsis blight	*Phomopsis vexans*
6.	Powdery mildew	*Erysiphe cichoracearum*

CUCURBITS

1.	Anthracnose	*Collectotrichum lagenarium*
2.	Downy mildew	*Pseudoperonospora cubensis*
3.	Powdery mildew	*Erysiphe cichoracearum*
4.	Leaf spot	*Cercospora citronella*
5.	Mosaic	*Marmor cucmeris* var. *vulgare*
6.	Wilt	*Erwinia tracheiphila*

CHILLIES

1.	Damping off	*Pythium aphanidermatum*
2.	Fruit-rot and Die-back	*Colletotrichum capsici*
3.	Alternaria Fruit-rot	*Alternaria solani*
4.	Cercospora leaf spot	*Cercospora capsici*
5.	Powdery mildew	*Leveillula taurica*
6.	Wilt	*Fusarium oxysporum* f.*solani*
7.	Bacterial leaf spot	*Xanthomonas campestris* p.v. *vesicatoria*
8	Mosaic	TMV and PVY
9.	Leaf curl	Tobacco leaf curl virus

Sl.No.	Common Name	Name of the Pathogen

CRUCIFERS

1.	Club root	*Plasmodiophora brassicae*
2.	Downy mildew	*Peronospora parasitica*
3.	Black leaf spot	*Alternaria brassicae*
4.	White blister	*Albugo candida*
5.	Stalk rot	*Sclerotinia sclerotiorum*
6.	Black leg	*Phoma lingam*
7.	Black rot	*Xanthomonas campestris* pv. *campestris*

BEAN

1.	Anthracnose	*Colletotrichum lindemuthianum*
2.	Powdery mildew	*Erysiphe polygoni*
3.	Rust	*Uromyces phaseoli typica*
4.	Leaf spot	*Cercospora cruenta*
5.	Mosaic	*Phaseolus virus*
6.	Yellow mosaic	*Bean yellow mosaic virus*

PEAS

1.	Powdery mildew	*Erysiphe polygoni*
2.	Downy mildew	*Peronospora pisi*
3.	Leaf blight	*Ascochyta pisi*
4.	Wilt	*Fusarium oxysporum* f.sp.*pisi*
5.	Rust	*Uromyces fabae*
6.	Bacterial blight	*Pseudomonas syringae* pv. *syringae*

Diseases of Tuber Crops

Sl.No.	Common Name	Name of the Pathogen

POTATO

1.	Early blight	*Alternaria solani*
2.	Late blight	*Phytophthora infestans*
3.	Blackscurf or stem canker	*Rhizoctonia solani*
4.	Brown rot Wilt (or) Ring diseases	*Pseudomonas solanacearum race*
5.	Wart	*Synchytrium endobioticum*

Sl.No.	Common Name	Name of the Pathogen
COLOCASIA		
1.	Phytophthora Blight	*Phytophthora colocasiae*
SUGARBEAT		
1.	Cercospora Leaf Spot	*Cercospora beticola*
2.	Phoma Leaf Spot and Root Rot	*Phoma betae*
3.	Rhizoctonia Dry Rot	*Rhizoctonia solani*
RADISH		
1.	Damping off	*Pythium aphanidermatum*
2.	White rust	*Albugo candida*
3.	Leaf spot	*Alternaria brassicae*
YAM		
1.	Root rot	*Rhizoctonia solani*

Post-harvest Diseases of Fruits

Sl.No.	Common Name	Name of the Pathogen
Mango		
1.	Anthracnose	*Colletotrichum gloeosporioides*
2.	Black Mould Rot	*Aspergillus niger*
3.	Soft Rot	*Rhizopus arrhizus*
4.	Stem End Rot	*Diplodia natalensis*
5.	Fruit Rot of **Banana**	*Botryodiplodia theobromae*
6.	Fruit Rot of **Citrus**	*Penicillium italicum*
7.	Fruit Rot of **Guava**	*Phoma psidii., Macrophomina allababadensis, Phytophthora.*
8.	Fruit Rot of **Payaya**	*Rhizopus stolonifier, Macrophomina phaseoli, Phomopsis caricae-papayae*
9.	Stem End Rot of **Pineapple**	*Ceratocystis paradoxa*
Pome and Sone fruits		
10.	Core rot	*Alternaria alternate*
11.	Grey Mould Rot	*Botryotinia fuckeliana*
12.	Bitter Rot	*Glomerella cingulata, Gloeosporium fructigenum.*
13.	Rhizopus Rot	*Rhizopus stolonifer, Rhizopus arrhizus*
14.	Blue Mould Rot	*Penicillium expansum*
15.	Phytophthors Fruit Rot	*Phytophthora cactorum, P. syringae*

Nematode Diseases of Temperate Fruits

Nematode Diseases of Tropical and Sub-Tropical fruits

Sl.No.	Common Name	Name of the Pathogen
Major Nematode pests		
1.	Root-Knot Nematodes	*Meloidogyne incognita, Meloidogyne indica, Meloidogyne javanica*
2.	Reniform Nematodes	*Rotylenchulus reniformist*
3.	Citrus Nematodes	*Tylenchulus semipenetrans*
4.	Burrowing Nematode	*Radepholus similes*
5.	Lesion Nematode	*Pratylenchus coffeae*
6.	Spiral Nematode	*Helicotylenchus multicinctus*
7.	Lance Nematode	*Hoplolaimus indicus,*
8.	Cyst Nematode	*Heterodera oryzicola*

Nematode Diseases of Vegetables

Sl.No.	Common Name	Name of the Pathogen
Cyst		
1.	Root-Knot	*Meloidogyne* spp
2.	Potato Cyst	Globodera rostochienensis
3.	Reniform	*Rotylenchulus reniformis*
4.	Root Lesion	*Pratylenchus* spp
5.	Stunt	*Tylenchorhynchus* spp
6.	Stem, Bulb	*Ditylenchus dipsaci*

Storage Disease of Vegetables

Sl.No.	Common Name	Name of the Pathogen
1.	Bacterial Soft Rot	*Erwinia caratovora* pv. *carotovora*
2.	Rhizopus Soft Rot	*Rhizopus* spp.
3.	Grey Mould	*Botrysis cinerea* Fr., *B. allii*
4.	Dry Rot of Potato	*Fusarium trichothecioides, F. solani* f.sp. *radicicola*
5.	Pink Rot	*Phytophthora erythroseptica*

Ornamental Plants

Sl.No.	Common Name	Name of the Pathogen
ANTHURIUM		
1.	Bacterial wilt	*Raostonia solanacearum*
2.	Bacterial blight	*Xanthomonas campestris* cv. *dieffenbachiae*
3.	Anthracnose	*Gloemerella cingulata*
4.	Balck rot and leaf blight	*Phytophthora nicotianae* var. *parasitica* and *P. citrophthora*
CARNATION		
1.	Wilt	*Fusarium oxysporum* f.sp. *dianthi*
2.	Foot rot	*Phytophthora* sp., *Pythium* sp., *Rhixoctonia solani*, *Sclerotinia slcerotiarum*
3.	Basal rot	*Sclerotium rolfsii*
4.	Leaf spot	*Alternaria dianthi*
5.	Bacterial wilt	*Pseudomonas caryophylli*
6.	Viral diseases	Transmitted by mize (Vector)
CHINA ASTER		
1.	Collar and root rot	*Phytophthora cryptogea*
2.	Wilt	*Fusarium* spp.
CHRYSANTHEMUM		
1.	Wilt	*Fusarium oxysporum* f.sp. *chrysanthemi*
2.	Stem rot	*Fusarium solani*
3.	Root rot	*Pythium* sp. and *Phytophthora* sp.
4.	Bacterial blight	*Erwinia chrysanthemi*
5.	Powdery mildew	*Oidium chrysanthemi*
6.	Leaf spot and flower blight	*Alternaria* sp., *Septoria chrysanthemella*
8.	Viroid disease	*Chrysanthemum* stunt viroid
CROSSANDRA		
1.	Foot and root rot	*Phytophthora nicotianae*
2.	Flower blight	*Alternaria* sp.
GERBERA		
1.	Foot rot	*Phytophthora cryptogea*
2.	Wilt	*Fusarium oxysporum* f.sp. *dianthi*
3.	Blight or grey mold	*Botrytis cinerea*

Sl.No.	Common Name	Name of the Pathogen
4.	Root rot	*Pythium* sp*Sclerotiumrolfsii, Rhixoctonia solani*
5.	Powdery mildew	*Erysiphe cichoracearum, Oidium crysiphoides* f.sp. *gerbera*
6.	Phyllody	*Phytoplasmas*

GLADIOLUS

1.	Wilt	*Fusarium oxysporum* f.sp. *gladioli*
2.	Neck rot	*Pseudomonas marginata, Stromatinia gladioli, Botrytis gladidorum*
3.	Corn rot	*Fusarium, Curvularia, Stromatinia, Botrytis and Penecillium* spp.
4.	Viral diseases	
5.	Aster yellows	MLOs

JASMINE

1.	Leaf spot	*Cercospora jasminicola, Alternaria jasmine, A. alternate*
2.	Rust	*Uromyces hobsoni*

MARIGOLD

1.	Wilt and stem rot	*Phytophthora cryptogea*
2.	Collar and root rot	*Pellicularia filamentosa, P. rolfsii, Pythium ultimum, Sclerotinia slerotiarum*
3.	Leaf spot and blight	*Alternaria* sp., *Septoria* sp., *Cercospora* sp.
4.	Powdery mildew	*Oidium* sp., *Leveillula taurica*

ORCHIDS

1.	Leaf spot	*Gloeosporium Cercospora, Colletotrichum* and *Phyllostictina*
2.	*Pythium* rot	*Phythium ultinum*
3.	Heart rot	*Phytophthora palmivora*
4.	Flower blight	*Botrytis cinerea*

ROSE

1.	Powdery mildew	*Sphaerotheca pannosa*
2.	Black spot	*Diplocarpon rosae*
3.	Die-back	*Diplodia rosarum, Colletotrichum* sp.
4.	Downy mildew	*Pernospora sparsa*
5.	Grey mold	*Botrytis cinerea*

Sl.No.	Common Name	Name of the Pathogen
6.	Rust	*Phragmidium* spp.
7.	Rose mosaic	*Phyllocoptes fructiphylus*
8.	Crown gall	*Agrobacterium tumefaciens*
TUBEROSE		
1.	Basal rot	*Sclerotium rolfsii*
2.	Flower blight	*Botrytis elliptica*

Medicinal Plants

Sl.No.	Common Name	Name of the Pathogen
ASGANDH		
1.	Seedling-rot	*Fusarium* sp. *Rhizoctonia* sp. *Pythium* sp.
2.	Leaf blight	*Alternaria tenuis*
3.	Die-back	*Colletotrichum* sp.
4.	Myrothecium leaf spot	*Myrothecium roridum*
5.	Virus disease	Tobacco leaf-curl virus
***CHLOROPHYTUM* SP.**		
1.	Anthracnose	*Colletorichum* sp.
2.	Chlorosis	*Ferrous deficiency*
GLYCYRRHIZA GLABRA		
1.	Leaf spot	*Cercospora cavarae*
2.	Powdery mildew	*Laveillula taurica L. leguminosarum Oidiopsistaurica*
3.	Rust	*Uromyces glycyrrhizae*
ISABGOL		
1.	Damping-off	*Pythium ultimum Rhizoctonia solani*
2.	Wilt	*F. solani, F.oxysporum*
3.	Downy mildew	*Peronospora alta, P. plantaginis*
4.	Powdery mildew	*Erysiphe cichoracearum*
5.	Leaf blight	*Alternaria alternate*
OPIUM POPPY		
1.	Downy mildew	*Peronospora arborescens*
2.	Powdery mildew	*Erysiphe polygoni*
3.	Root rot	*Sclerotinia sclerotiorum, Macrophomina phaseolina, Rhizoctonia sp, Fusarium semiitectum*

Sl.No.	Common Name	Name of the Pathogen
4.	Capsule infection	*Macrosporium paraveris, Allernaria brassicae* var. *somniferum, A. alternate, Dendryphion penicillatum*
5.	Mosaic	*Turnip mosaic virus*
6.	Broomrape	*Orobanche papaveris*

PERIWINKLE

1.	Blight	*Phytophthora* sp.

SARPAGANDHA

1.	Wilt	*Fusarium oxysporum* var. *serpentine*
2.	Powdery mildew	*Leveillula taurica*
3.	Leaf blight and bud rot	*Alternaria tenuis*
4.	Leaf spot	*Cerospora rauvolfiae*
5.	Mosaic	Tobacco mosaic virus (TMV)
6.	Phyllody	Yellow virus

SENNA

1.	Leaf spot	*Alternaria alternate*
2.	Damping-off at seedling stage	*Rhizoctonia bataticola*

Aromatic Plants

Sl.No.	Common Name	Name of the Pathogen

MENTHA ARVENSIS* VAR. *PIPERESCENS

1.	Wilt	*Verticillium alboatrum*
2.	Stolon-rot	*Rhizoctonia bataticola, Macrophomina phaseoli, Thielavia basicola*
3.	Sclerotium-rot	*Sclerotium rolfsii*
4.	Powdery mildew	*Erysiphe cichoracearum*
5.	Leaf spot	*Curvularia lunata*
6.	Leaf blight	*Alternaria* sp.
7.	Rust	*Puccinia menthae*
8.	Red leaf-spot	*Colletotrichum graminicola,C. condatum*
9.	Leaf blight	*Curvulaia evagrostidis, C. verruciformis, C.trofoli, C. andropogonis*
10.	Eye leaf-spot	*Helmin-thosporium sacchari H-leucostylum (drecheslera victoriae, D. holmi)*

11.	Rust	*Puccinia nakanishikii*
12.	Smut	*Tolyposporium christensenii*
13.	Wilt	*Fusarium moniliformae (Gibberella fujikuroi)*

VETIVER (khus)

1.	Leaf blight	*Curvularia trifolii*
2.	Gloeocercospora leaf spot	*Gloeocercospora*
3.	Helminthosporium leaf spot	*Helminthosporium* sp.
4.	Smut	*Ustilago vetiveriae*

Plantation Crops

Sl.No.	Common Name	Name of the Pathogen
ARECANUT		
1.	Fruit rot	*Phytophthora palmivora*
2.	Foot rot	*Ganordema lucidum*
CASHEW NUT		
1.	Inflorescence blight	*Gloeosporium mangiferae/Phomopsis anacaradii/ Fusarium* sp.
2.	Die-back or pink disease	*Corticum salminicolor (Pellicularia salmonicolori)*
3.	Damping-off seedlings	*Fusarium* spp., *Phythium* spp., *Phytophthora palmivora* spp., *Cylindrocladium scoparium*
4.	Anthracnose	*Colletotrichum gloeosporioides*
COCOA		
1.	Black-pod	*Phytophthora palmivora*
2.	Canker	*Phytophthora palmivora*
3.	Charcoal pod rot	*Botryodiplodia theobromae*
4.	White thread blight	*Marasmius scandens*
5.	Vascular streak die-back	*Oncobasidium theobromoe*
6.	Pink disease	*Pellicularia salmonicolor*
COCONUT		
1.	Bud rot	*Phytophthora palmivora*
2.	Stem bleeding	*Thielaviopsis paradoxa*
3.	Wilt	*Ganoderma applanatum, Ganoderma lucidum*
4.	Grey leaf spot/blight	*Pestalotia palmarium*

Sl.No.	Common Name	Name of the Pathogen
TEA		
1.	Blister blight	*Exobasidium vexans*
2.	Grey blight	*Pestalotia theae*
3.	Sooty mould	*Capnodium* sp.
COFFEE		
1.	Rust	*Hemileia vastatrix*
2.	Anthracnose	*Glomerella cingulata*
3.	Brown eye spot	*Cercospora coffeicola*
4.	Soty mould	*Capnodium brasiliense*
OIL PALM		
1.	Spear-rot	*Phytoplasma*
2.	Fruit-rot	*Marasmium palmivorus*
3.	Bud-rot	*Ermima* sp.
RUBBER		
1.	Abnormal Leaf Fall and Stem Rot	*Phytophthora palmivora*
2.	Powdery Mildew	*Oidium heveae*

Diseases of Species

Sl.No.	Common Name	Name of the Pathogen
BETELVINE		
1.	Wilt or root-rot	*Phytophthora parasitica var piperina*
2	Powdery mildew	*Oidium piperis*
3.	Leaf spot	*Colletotrichum* sp.
4.	Wilt	*Sclerotium rolfsii*
CARDAMOM		
1.	Mosaic or Katte disease of small Cardamom	Cardamom mosaic virus
2.	Nilgiri Necrosis disease	Necrosis virus
3.	Vein-clearing	Vein-clearing virus
4.	Mosaic or Chirke disease of large Cardamom	Chirke virus
5.	Foorkey disease	Foorkey virus

Sl.No.	Common Name	Name of the Pathogen
CUMIN		
1.	Cumin Wilt	*Fusarium oxysporum* f. sp. *Cumini*
2.	Powdery Mildew	*Erysiphe polygoni*
3	Blight	*Alternaria burnsii*
CORIANDER		
1.	Stem Gall	*Protomyces macrosporus*
2.	Root Rot	*Phytophthora nicotianae* var. *parasitica, Rhizoctonia* spp.
3.	Leaf Spot	*Alternaria* spp.
4.	Wilt	*Fusarium oxysporum* f.sp. *corianderii*
5.	Powdery Mildew	*Erysiphe polygoni*
FENNEL		
1.	Powdery Mildew	*Leveillula taurica*
2.	Leaf Spot	*Cercosporidium punctum,*
3.	Blight	*Ramularia foeniculi*
FENUGREEK		
1.	Powdery Mildew	*Erysiphe polygone, Leveillula taurica*
2.	Root Rot	*Rhizoctonia solani*
GINGER		
1.	Leaf spot	*Phyllosticta zingiberi*
2.	Soft rot	*Pythium aphanidermatumor, P.graminicolum*
NUTMEG		
1.	Thread blight	*Marasmius pulcherima, M.equicrinus*
PEPPER		
1.	Leaf spot	*Collectotrichum* sp.
2.	Red rust	*Cephaleuros* sp.
3.	Quick wilt	*Phytophthora capsici*
TURMERIC		
1.	Leaf spot	*Colletotricchum capsici*
2.	Rhizome rot	*Pythium graminicolum*
3.	Leaf blotch	*Taphrina maculans*
VANILLA		
1.	Wilt	*Fusarium oxysporum*

Glossary

Abiotic: Pertaining to physical and inorganic components. For example, diseases/disorders in plants can be caused by abiotic factors such as extremes of heat, light, moisture, lack of nutrients etc.

Appressorium (pl. Appressoria): An enlarged fungal filament that adheres to the surface of the host, prior to penetration.

Avirulent: Unable to cause disease, lacking virulence (see virulent); non-pathogenic.

Biotic: ertaining to life and therefore living organisms. For example, plant diseases of a biotic origin are caused by living organisms such as insects, nematodes, etc.

Biotroph: An organism that can live and reproduce only on another living organism. A biotroph is completely dependent on the host organism as a source of nutrients, *i.e.*, it is an obligate parasite. Compare with necrotroph.

Blight: A disease characterized by rapid and widespread death of plant tissue. Blight may take the form of extensive spotting, discoloration, wilting, or destruction of leaves, flowers and stems.

Cultivar: A cultivated plant variety or cultural selection; a plant type within a species that has recognizable characteristics as a result of deliberate genetic manipulation. Distinguishable characteristics may include colour, flower shape, fruits, seeds and height.

Cuticle: The waxy or fatty layer covering epidermal cells of plant surfaces exposed to air such as leaves, stems and fruit. The cuticle is water-repellent and aids the plant in conserving water by reducing the amount of water vapour lost to the air from plant surfaces, particularly the upper surface of leaves. In zoology, cuticle also refers to the non-cellular outer layer of an insect or a nematode.

Damping off: The collapse and rot of seedlings near soil level before emergence or soon after emergence. Damping off is caused by fungi: *Pythium* spp., *Fusarium* spp., and *Rhizoctonia* spp.

Defensins: Antimicrobial proteins that inhibit the growth and development of pathogens. Plant defenses are found throughout the plant kingdom and are released upon seed germination, creating an antimicrobial environment around the seed while it germinates.

Dieback: Progressive death of shoots, and branched roots, sometimes even leading to complete death of the plant.

Disease: Any malfunctioning of host cells and tissues that results from continuous irritation by a pathogenic agent or environmental factor which leads to the development of symptoms; abnormal functioning of physiological processes of an organism.

Disease Incidence: The number of plants affected by a disease within a population.

Disease Severity: The measure of damage done by a disease.

Ectoparasite: A parasite that lives and feeds from the exterior of its host's cells or tissues. Compare with endoparasite.

Endobiotic: Describes an organism living within the cells or tissues of a host organism. Endobiotic organisms are endoparasites.

Epiphytic: Living on the surface of a plant, but not as a parasite and without causing infection.

Eradication: The control of plant disease by eliminating the pathogen after it is established or by eliminating all of the plants that carry the pathogen.

Exclusion: A method of disease prevention in which the pathogen or infected plant material is excluded from crop production areas. (See quarantine).

Extracellular: Outside a cell.

Fungicide: A substance (chemical or physical) that kills or inhibits the growth of fungi.

Gall: An abnormal growth or swelling produced as a result of pathogenic invasion.

Genotype: The genetic make-up of an individual or group.

Gum: Gelatinous, sugary substance that is synthenized and secreted by plant tissues.

Haustorium (pl. Haustoria): A specialized branch of a fungal hypha formed inside a living cell of the host plant in order to obtain nutrients.

Hemibiotroph: A parasite that initially forms an association with living cells of the host, much like a biotroph, and then in the later stages of infection it becomes necrotrophic, actively killing host cells.

Host: An organism harbouring a parasite or pathogen.

Host Range: The range of plants on which an organism feeds, particularly a parasite; the range of plants in which a pathogen is capable of causing disease.

Hydathode: A specialized epidermal leaf structure with one or more openings through which water is discharged from the leaf interior to its surface.

Hypersensitive: The state of being extremely or excessively sensitive. It often refers to an extreme reaction by a plant to an invading pathogen in which the plant tissue around infected sites dies in order to prevent further spread of the infection.

Hypha (pl. Hyphae): A single tubular thread-like filament of a fungal mycelium. The hypha is the basic structural unit of a fungus.

Inoculate: To introduce a microorganism or virus into an environment (*i.e.*, an organism or culture medium) suitable for its growth; to insert a pathogen into healthy tissue.

Inoculum (pl. Inocula): A pathogen or its parts which can cause infection when transferred to a favorable location; the population of microorganisms introduced in an inoculation.

Latent Infection: Where the host is infected with a pathogen but does not show any symptoms.

Lignin: A complex polymer deposited in some cell walls of vascular plants. Lignin is one of the main constituents of secondary walls and wood. It gives compressive strength and rigidity to the cell walls as well as making it impermeable to water.

Mosaic: Patchy variation of normal green colour in leaves, usually light and dark green mosaic, symptomatic of many viral diseases.

Mycelium (pl. Mycelia): A mass of hyphae that forms the body (thallus) of a fungus.

Multigene Family: A set of genes that, due to their high degree of sequence similarity, are believed to have evolved from a single ancestral gene.

Necrosis: The death of cells, often accompanied by black or brown darkening of the tissue.

Necrotroph: An organism (parasite) that causes the death of host tissues as it grows through them, obtaining its energy from the dead cells. Compare with biotroph.

Obligate Parasite: An organism that is only capable of living as a parasite in association with its host plant. The term is synonymous with biotroph.

Parasite: An organism or virus living in or on another organism (host) from which it obtains its nutrient supply. A parasite is not necessarily a pathogen.

Parenchyma: The soft tissue comprised of living, thin-walled cells of variable size and form, Parenchyma cells are the most abundant cell type in plants. In leaves, parenchyma is differentiated into two forms:

Palisade parenchyma: the tissue found beneath the upper epidermis of leaves, composed of elongate, tubular cells aligned perpendicular to the leaf surface. Palisade parenchyma cells generally contain an abundance of chloroplasts.

Spongy parenchyma: the tissue typically found between the palisade parenchyma and the lower epidermis of leaves. Spongy parenchyma consists of loosely arranged, irregularly-shaped cells containing chloroplasts and is interspersed with intercellular spaces.

Pathogen: A disease causing organism or agent.

Pathogenesis: The sequence of processes in disease development that describes a pathogen's association with its host. The sequence begins with initial contact between the pathogen and host and ends when the pathogen is no longer associated with that host (*i.e.*, when the host/pathogen dies or the pathogen moves to another host).

Pathogenicity: The ability to cause disease.

Penetration: Initial invasion of a host by pathogen.

Penetration Peg: A structure found in some plant parasitic fungi. The penetration peg is a specialized, narrow, hyphal strand located on the underside of an appressorium that penetrates the epidermal cell wall.

Phenotype: The visible physical characteristics of an organism determined by the interaction of its genotype with the environment.

Phloem: The food-conducting and food-storing tissue in the roots, stems, and leaves of vascular plants.

Photosynthesis: The production of carbohydrates from carbon dioxide and water in the presence of chlorophyll(s), using light energy and releasing oxygen as a by-product.

Phytoalexin: A substance produced in higher plants in response to a number of stimuli (chemical, physical or biological) that inhibits the development of a microorganism.

Phytoplasmas: Phloem-dwelling prokaryotic microorganisms, transmitted by phloem-feeding insects.

Powdery Mildew: White powdery 'bloom' on the plant surface caused by the production of fungal mycelium, conidiophores and conidia by members of the *Erysiphales* (powdery mildew fungi).

Primary Inoculum: Inoculum that initiates disease in the field following a dormant stage in its life cycle (called over-wintering or over-summering). Compare with secondary inoculum.

Propagules: Any part of an organism capable of independent growth (*e.g.*, a spore, a mycelial fragment, etc.).

Protectant: Any chemical agent that interacts with a pathogen on the plant surface to prevent infection.

Protectant fungicide: A protectant that kills or inhibits the growth of fungi. See fungicide.

Pustule: A blister-like spore mass breaking through a plant epidermics.

Pleiotropic: Having multiple effects.

Proteinaceous: Of or related to protein.

Quarantine: Legal restriction of the transport of plants and/or plant parts in order to prevent the spread of pests and pathogens. In order to accomplish this plants may be held in isolation (*i.e.*, quarantine) for an extended period of time to ensure that they are free of pests and diseases.

Race: A subgroup of pathogens within a species that infect a given set of plant varieties. Races may be distinguished from each other by virulence or symptom expression but not by morphology.

Resistant: Possessing qualities that prevent or impede the development of a disease.

Resistance: The power of an organism to exclude or overcome, completely or partially, the effects of a pathogen or some other damaging factor.

Respiration: An intracellular process which consists of a series of chemical reactions that make energy available through the oxidation of carbohydrates, fats and proteins. This process produces carbon dioxide and water as by-products and is termed aerobic respiration because it uses oxygen (although the initial stages of the process are anaerobic, *i.e.*, do not require oxygen).

Resting Spore: A thick-walled spore, usually formed by a sexual process, that germinates after remaining in a dormant state for an extended period of time.

Rot: The disintegration of tissue, often caused by enzyme or toxins produced by pathogens.

Rust: Rust-coloured pustules formed by members of the *Uredinales* (rust fungi).

Saprophyte: An organism that obtains nourishment from non-living organic matter (usually dead and decaying plant or animal matter) by absorbing soluble organic compounds.

Scab: A discrete, superficial roughened lesion.

Sclerotium (pl. Sclerotia): A hard, resistant vegetative resting body of a fungus composed of a compact mass of hyphae and capable of surviving under unfavorable environmental conditions. Under favorable conditions, the sclerotium can produce sexual or asexual fruiting bodies.

Secondary Inoculum: Inoculum produced by infections that took place during the same growing season. Compare with primary inoculum.

Secondary Metabolite: A compound that is not necessary for growth or maintenance of cellular functions but is, in general, synthesized for the protection of a cell or microorganism during the stationary phase of its growth cycle. In plants, secondary metabolites are believed to be important in the attraction of pollinators and to have a function in defense, as some metabolites have antimicrobial properties. Also known as secondary products.

Smut: A disease characterized by black spore masses on leaves, stems or inflorescences, caused by members of the *ustilaginales* (smut fungi).

Sporangiophore: Sporangium-bearing body of a fungus.

Sporangium (pl. Sporangia): A unicellular or multicellular sac-like structure in fungi that produces asexual spores.

Spore: A specialized reproductive body in fungi (and some other organisms), containing one or more cells, capable of developing into an adult.

Stoma (pl. Stomata): A minute opening in the epidermis of leaves and stems through which gasses pass. The stoma is bordered by two guard cells which open and close depending on their turgidity. The term stoma is often used to refer to the entire stomatal apparatus, *i.e.*, the guard cells as well as the pore they surround.

Systemic: (1) pertaining to a disease in which the pathogen spreads generally throughout the plant; **(2)** pertaining to a chemical absorbed into the plant through root or foliage and transported internally throughout the plant.

Systemic fungicide: A chemical agent that spreads internally through the plant and eradicates established fungal infections. See fungicide.

Tillage: The process of turning or mixing the soil.

Toxin: In general, a poisonous substance of biological origin. Specifically, a compound produced by a microorganism which is toxic to other organisms.

Transcription: The process whereby a base sequence of messenger RNA (mRNA) is synthesized on a complementary segment of DNA.

Translation: The process that occurs at the ribosome whereby the information in messenger RNA (mRNA) is used to assemble amino acids into a protein.

Translocation: The long-distance transport of water, nutrients, chemicals, or food materials within a plant.

Transpiration: The loss of water vapour from leaf surfaces and other parts of the plant exposed to the air. Most transpiration occurs through stomata.

Tylose, Tylosis (pl. Tyloses): A balloon-like outgrowth from a parenchyma cell that expands through a pit in a xylem vessel wall and into the lumen of the vessel, either blocking it completely or partially.

Vascular: Pertaining to any plant tissue or region consisting of fluid-conducting tissue; for example, xylem and phloem. The term is also sometimes applied to a pathogen that grows primarily in the conducting tissues of the plant.

Vascular Wilt: A disease in which the pathogen is confined to the vascular system of the host and in which wilting is a characteristic symptom; plants lose their turgidity and become flaccid, leaves collapse.

Vector: Any living organism (*e.g.*, insect, mite, bird, nematode, parasitic plant, human, etc.) that transmits a pathogen from an infected organism to an uninfected one.

Virulence: The degree or measure of pathogenicity of a given pathogen; relative capacity to cause disease.

Virulent: Strongly pathogenic; capable of causing severe disease (see avirulent).

Virus: A submicroscopic, non-cellular structure consisting of a core of infectious nucleic acid (either RNA or DNA) within a protein coat.

Xylem: A complex vascular tissue through which water and minerals are conducted through the plant. Xylem also aids in the structural support of a plant as the primary component of its cell walls is lignin.

Yellows: plant disease characterized by yellowing and stunting of the plant.

References

1. Wikipedia, The Free Encyclopedia, www.wikipedia.org.

2. J.G. Manners. 1993. Principles of Plant Pathology, 2 Edition. Cambridge University Press, Cambridge, UK. 343 p.

3. Agrios, George N. 2005. Plant Pathology. Fifth Edition. Academic Press, New York. 922p.

4. Walker, J.C. 1972. Plant Pathology. Third Edition. Tata McGraw Hill. 819p.

5. Strange, Richard N. 2003. Introduction to Plant Pathology. John Wiley, West Sussex, England. 464p.

6. www.fungionline.org.uk/3hyphae/1hypha_ultra.html

7. www.slic2.wsu.edu:82/../pages/Chap3.html

8. www.apsnet.org/online/feature/huanglongbing

9. www.jic.ac.uk/staff/saskia-hogenhout/default.html

10. www.answers.com/topic/spiroplasma

11. bakerlab.berkeley.edu/index.php?img=1

12. www.biologie.uni-hamburg.de/bzf/mppg/agviroid.htm

13. www.scielo.br/scielo.php?script=sci_arttext..

14. www.ctahr.hawaii.edu/nelsons/Misc/

15. www.ctahr.hawaii.edu/nelsons/Misc/

16. www.apsnet.org/online/feature/milestones/

17. www.humboldt.edu/~dll2/358/slime/protist.html

18. www.vgavic.org.au/vegetables-victoria-researc..

19. www.bsu.edu/classes/ruch/msa/barr.html

20. vegetablemdonline.ppath.cornell.edu/diagnosti..

21. botit.botany.wisc.edu/toms_fungi/mar2001.html

22. www.apsnet.org/../Images/potatolateblight.htm

23. ipm.illinois.edu/../series700/rpd705/index.html

24. www.omafra.gov.on.ca/../crops/facts/90-125.htm

25. www.mycolog.com/chapter2b.htm

26. www.answers.com/topic/rhizopus

27. www.ctahr.hawaii.edu/nelsons/papaya/papaya.html

28. www.plante-doktor.dk/meldug.htm

29. www.bayercropscience.bg/../BG_Vine_program_p_2

30. ipmnet.org/plant-disease/disease.cfm?RecordID=525

31. www.apsnet.org/online/archive/1998/rust044.htm and teapotshappen. wordpress.com/../

32. www.ces.ncsu.edu/../index.html; b) ipm.illinois.edu/../series300/rpd303/ index.html;

c) extension.missouri.edu/publications/DisplayPu..

33. vegetablemdonline.ppath.cornell.edu/PhotoPage..; and www.extension.umn. edu/../YGLN-Aug0104.html

34. www.potatodiseases.org/earlyblight.html

35. www.rbgsyd.nsw.gov.au/../Sclerotium

36. www.hdc.org.uk/herbs/page.asp?id=15

37. www.doacs.state.fl.us/pi/canker/

38. www.treehelp.com/trees/crabapple/trees-diseas..

39. www.caf.wvu.edu/../viskeyargu.htm

40. www.cals.ncsu.edu/course/pp728/Ralstonia/Toma..

41. www.usask.ca/../vegetable/definition.htm

42. http://www.ncbi.nlm.nih.gov/ICTVdb/ICTVdB/

43. www.apsnet.org/../Activities/TMV/text/fig01.htm

44. www.veksthus.no/hovedsiden.html

45. www.inra.fr/hyp3/pathogene/6beyevi.htm

46. www.plantmanagementnetwork.org/../2007/kenaf/

47. www.indianjournals.com/ijor.aspx?target=ijor:..

48. www.freshplaza.com/news_detail.asp?id=9853

49. ·www.takestan.mihanblog.com/post/272

50. vegetablemdonline.ppath.cornell.edu/PhotoPage..

51. photos.eppo.org/index.php/image/1950-csvd00-0..

52. susveg-asia.nri.org/susvegasiabrinjalipm4.html

53. pbin.nbii.org/reportapest/pestlist/bbtv.htm

54. www.eppo.org/../virus/PSTVd/PSTVD0_images.htm

55. forums.gardenweb.com/../msg0308103831085.html

56. flickr.com/photos/dinesh_valke/3272190770/

57. www.ikisan.com/links/ap_tobaccoDisease per cent 20Mana..

58. www.parasiticplants.siu.edu/Scrophulariaceae/..

Index